DOING PRACTICE-BASED RESEARCH *in* THERAPY

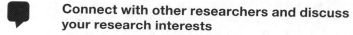
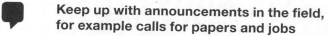
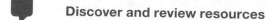
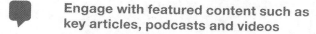
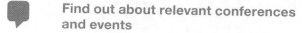
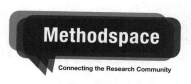
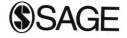

A REFLEXIVE APPROACH

DOING PRACTICE-BASED
RESEARCH *in* THERAPY

SOFIE BAGER-CHARLESON

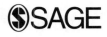

Los Angeles | London | New Delhi
Singapore | Washington DC

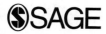

SAGE

Los Angeles | London | New Delhi
Singapore | Washington DC

SAGE Publications Ltd
1 Oliver's Yard
55 City Road
London EC1Y 1SP

SAGE Publications Inc.
2455 Teller Road
Thousand Oaks, California 91320

SAGE Publications India Pvt Ltd
B 1/I 1 Mohan Cooperative Industrial Area
Mathura Road
New Delhi 110 044

SAGE Publications Asia-Pacific Pte Ltd
3 Church Street
#10-04 Samsung Hub
Singapore 049483

Editor: Kate Wharton
Editorial assistant: Laura Walmsley
Production editor: Rachel Burrows
Marketing manager: Tamara Navaratnam
Cover design: Jennifer Crisp
Typeset by: C&M Digitals (P) Ltd, Chennai, India
Printed in Great Britain by Henry Ling Limited, at
The Dorset Press, Dorchester, DT1 1HD

Library of Congress Control Number: 2013941885

British Library Cataloguing in Publication data

A catalogue record for this book is available from the
British Library

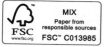

MIX
Paper from
responsible sources
FSC™ C013985
www.fsc.org

ISBN 978-1-4462-6672-4
ISBN 978-1-4462-6673-1 (pbk)

Contents

About the author

Sofie Bager-Charleson is a psychotherapist, supervisor and writer. She draws from psychoanalytic, existential and cognitive behavioural theory with a particular interest in postmodern influences on therapy. She holds a PhD from Lund University in Sweden, where she specialised in attachment issues within families and reflective practice among teachers. She writes both fiction and non-fiction. She works as an academic adviser for psychotherapists on the work-based doctorate programme, DPsych with Metanoia/Middlesex University. She runs workshops and courses in therapeutic practice, reflective and creative writing, in both Sweden and England.

Preface

Learning how to use oneself creatively and effectively in the treatment process is an important aspect of psychotherapy. While emphasised in training for clinical practice, this level of self-awareness is often neglected in research about mental health. Research tends to be construed as something separate to ourselves and our daily lives; it is still commonly perceived as something which people in white coats do in laboratory-like circumstances. This book aims to demystify research, and will provide a step-by-step account with references to real-life research. The book links practical research skills to reflexivity. Reflexive awareness involves a deliberate attempt to position oneself as researcher in a linguistic, cultural, theoretical and personal context with potential biases and blind spots in mind. A significant feature for practice-based research is that it is situated in offices, hospitals and other real-life settings. It is never conducted in a vacuum; the purpose with practice-based research is often to include this 'messiness' of life. What is it like *really* to work in a ward with people suffering from dementia? What happens between staff and patients in their everyday meetings? What is it like to be staff, and to be a patient? How do the experiences differ between different individuals, and why?

The practice-based researcher listens out to everything from the most basic experience, such as the experience of attending others to the toilet, to more complex, organisational concerns. By learning more about everyday experiences in wards, schools and the psychotherapists' consultation rooms, the practice-based researcher hopes to contribute with a holistic approach to improvements. The way that practice-based researchers approach clients or patients in the context of different relationships and systems is carried through into the way they position themselves in their research. Their relationship with the research participants will be referred to as a significant conduit for the outcome. We will look at examples of how researchers pay careful attention both with regard to how their participants and interviewees perceive them, but also how they themselves are impacted by their participants. Seemingly small and mundane reactions, responses and findings are often attended to as significant features of the study. The impact that researchers and research participants may have on each other is, just like in therapeutic practice, carefully considered and assumed to impact the interviews, data analysis and general outcome of the study. The layout of the book runs as follows:

In **Chapter 1**, some key characteristics of practitioner research are explored. We will look at the role research may play in our everyday life and practice, for instance with reference to overlaps and differences between 'private' and 'public' research. The researcher as a person is at the forefront of **Chapter 2**. We will look at how prior personal and professional experiences may be integrated in our practice and research, for instance with regard to our choice of theory as well as our emotional responses to new situations. Methodological approaches play a crucial role in the layout and the outcome of our studies. We will look at the difference between quantitative and qualitative research, and also explore options for combining the two. In **Chapter 3**, Jean-Marc Dewaele and Beverley Costa illustrate this combination, and write about how mixed-methods became their chosen approach. Randomised controlled trials, systemic reviews and meta-analysis are some of the frequently used terms in today's research about therapy. In **Chapter 4** we will look closer into these concepts. Evidence-based research will be explored in more depth, and we will focus on the meaning and implications of a hierarchy of trustworthiness, with objectivity as an overarching aim. **Chapter 5** focuses on how to identify and articulate the research question. We will look at several different real-life examples and you will be encouraged to formulate a research question of your own. In **Chapter 6**, Simon du Plock writes about 'doing' a literature review and about how to critically engage with literature and research in your field. **Chapter 7** revolves around the ethical dimensions of research. The relationship between the researcher and research participants is typically close in practice-based research. These relationships will need to be carefully negotiated. We will explore some of the key differences and overlaps between research relationships and therapeutic relationships, and examine how we can prepare for the personal change and growth which both types of relationship tend to involve. The chapter includes examples of how to write research invitations and consent forms. **Chapter 8** pursues the focus on the relationship and its impact on the researcher and their research participants. We will look at examples where researchers consider their emotional responses with care, and take into account how their responses will impact on the way they meet, listen to and relate to their research participants. Emotional and unconscious processes will be explored in the context of reflective practice, and will be linked to the difference between espoused theory (the theory we are committed to) and our actual theory in action. **Chapter 9** revolves around the way that our epistemological stance may impact on the study. We will particularly explore the difference between realism, idealism and postmodern critique, and focus on the different approaches of subjectivity and objectivity in research. **Chapter 10** explores the meaning(s) of reflexivity. Practice-based research is never conducted in a vacuum. Underlying personal and cultural expectations, values and beliefs held by both the researcher and research participants are inevitable aspects of research conducted in real-life settings. In this chapter reflexivity is considered as ways of incorporating implicit, explicit, conscious and unconscious aspects of the research process without losing sight of scientific 'rigor'. Particular attention will be paid to what Finlay and Gough (2003) refer to as 'five variants' of reflexivity. **Chapter 11** looks at examples of research where reflexivity on introspection is adopted, for instance with reference to real-life examples of heuristic and autoethnographic research. **Chapter 12** looks at research where reflexivity focuses on intersubjective processes and reflections, for instance with reference to psychoanalytic research which puts transference, countertransference and 'unconscious' processes to the forefront. **Chapter 13** provides examples of research characterised by an emphasis on collaboration. For instance, we will look at real-life examples of co-operative inquiry into school-based therapy in socially deprived areas, and with reference to the role of black issues in counselling training. The chapter includes examples of how to invite people to join co-operative inquiry groups. Finally, in **Chapter 14**, Simon du Plock writes about the impacts of research and about ways of communicating our research findings with the outside world. **Chapter 15** offers some concluding remarks and reflections about the overall content of the book.

Acknowledgements

This book would never have been written without the contributors listed below. I am particularly grateful to **Simon du Plock**, who has contributed two chapters to this book. Simon is the Director of the Centre for Practice-Based Research and Head of the Post-Qualification Doctorates Department at the Metanoia Institute, London. His experiences from practice-based research have been invaluable.

I am also immensely grateful to Beverley and Jean-Marc for their contributions about research that is so close to my heart, and for their invaluable support at a vulnerable stage of the writing process. I am pleased to congratulate them for recently being awarded the BACP Equality and Diversity Award for their research. **Jean-Marc Dewaele** is Professor of Applied Linguistics and Multilingualism at Birkbeck, University of London. He researches individual differences in psycholinguistic, sociolinguistic, pragmatic, psychological and emotional aspects of Second Language Acquisition and Multilingualism. Dr **Beverley Costa** is a psychotherapist and the founder of Mothertongue, a multi-ethnic counselling service. She has been its director from its establishment in 2000 until the present day. Mothertongue provides a professional culturally and linguistically sensitive counselling service to people from the black and minority ethnic communities in their preferred language.

Another exceptionally inspirational friend and contributor is Dr **Marie Adams**. She is a psychotherapist, writer and works at the Metanoia Institute as a trainer. Marie's book, based on her research into the private lives of therapists, will be published later on this year. Thank you, too, to Dr **Stephen Adams-Langley**. He has worked in the voluntary sector for thirty years promoting the mental health of children and young people. His kindness, resilience and knowledge have found a home in school-based mental health programmes targeting hard-to-reach children who have been exposed to multiple risk factors for many years. Stephen has worked as a regional manager at Place2Be for sixteen years. Dr **Alan Priest** is another friend I want to thank. In this book, Alan shares examples from his innovative doctoral research about the relationship between change in clients' pronoun usage and outcomes in therapy. His study describes the impact of inviting clients to clients' 'own' experiences and emphasises how such interventions should be used with care.

I am grateful to Dr **Anne Atkinson**, who generously shares her valuable insights into the research process. Anne is a psychotherapist who originally carried out anthropological research. As a psychoanalytic psychotherapist with an insatiable spirit of inquiry, her research developed in new directions, as shown in this book. I am also immensely grateful to Dr **Maxine Daniels**, who has contributed for a second time to one of my books. Maxine brings fascinating insights into reflexivity in emotionally charged research settings. Maxine works as National Trainer with criminal justice agencies and as a Consultant and Supervisor in medium secure hospitals. **Pamela Stewart** has also contributed with invaluable insights and experiences. Her reflective infant-observations research in prison for the Tavistock Institute is referred to at several stages of this book. Pamela has worked in a Philadelphia Association therapeutic community and continues to work as a psychotherapist and supervisor in prisons as well as in private practice. Thank you, too, to **Stella Gould**, who works as a forensic psychotherapist with the Psychological Intelligence Foundation and who generously shares her experience of ethical procedures in difficult settings. Dr **Melanie Jo Hopkins Womble** also works as a psychotherapist in forensic settings. She recently completed her doctorate in Psychotherapy from Metanoia Institute which focused on 'staff experience of hope' with a view to developing the Forensic Recovery Model. Dr **Claire Asherson Bartram** is another former Metanoia student whose contribution is greatly appreciated. Claire works as Gestalt psychotherapist and group leader. Her doctoral project 'Narratives of mothers in stepfamily situations' interweaves her story as a mother with those of the women she interviewed. Thank you, too, to Dr **Roz D'Ombraine Hewitt**, who is a psychotherapist and trainer. Her experience of working in a psychiatric hospital inspired her first book, *Moving On: A Guide to Good Health and Recovery for People with a Diagnosis of Schizophrenia* (2007), and her doctoral research. **Guy Harrison** contributes with insightful reflections about methodology. Guy is a psychotherapist and an Anglican priest. He has worked for sixteen years at a senior level as a healthcare chaplain and counsellor within hospice, acute care and mental healthcare contexts. Dr **Lynne Souter-Anderson** shares her fascinating research journey, regarding her interest in the use of clay, arts and sand in therapy. She is the Director of the Bridging Creative Therapies Consultancy and offers workshops to all levels of practitioners nationally and internationally. **Rupert King** is currently undertaking a DPsych at Metanoia Institute and shares insightful reflections on the research process. He works as an existential psychotherapist in private practice and has taught on a number of Post-Graduate Diploma courses. I am also extremely grateful to Dr **Isha Mckenzie-Mavinga**, who contributes with so many important angles to contemporary research. Isha works as an integrative transcultural psychotherapist. She also lectures, supervises and has published several papers from her doctoral study on the process of understanding 'black issues' in counsellor training and practice.

I would like to thank Laura Walmsley, Kate Wharton, Luke Block and Alice Oven from Sage, for being so brilliant to work with. Thank you also to Mandy Kersey, our coordinator at Metanoia, for being such a kind and considerate friend.

Finally, I want to give a special thank-you to our children, Fina, Finbar and Leo. They have contributed to everything, from their kindness and inspiration to providing practical help. Fina contributed with editorial assistance and Finbar made abstract concepts digestible through graphics. Leo was there when I fell ill from a prolapsed disc in the neck during the project. I shall never forget! I also want to thank my husband Dermot for being my soul mate and for dancing with me in the office when my back injury threatened to return! Thank you, too, to my mother, Anna-Lena Bager, for always being so encouraging and supportive.

ONE   Real-life research

This chapter outlines the characteristics of practice-based research. We look at the role research may play in our everyday life, with reference to overlaps and differences between 'private' and 'public' research.

- Theory
- Interpretation
- Inductive and deductive reasoning
- Therapeutic modalities
- Countertransference, transference and projections
- Congruence
- Automatic thoughts

Introduction

Research plays a significant role in therapy today. From being steeped in mystery, psychotherapy has become a profession characterised by transparency and accountability. One of my favourite books during my own training was *The Analytic Experience* by Neville Symington. In it, Symington (1986: 9) boldly stated that 'it is as impossible to convey the sense of [psychotherapy] to another person, as it is to explain to an eight-year old child what it is like to be in love.' These kinds of comments seem out of place today. Ambiguities are giving way to 'evidence' and 'knowing'. Wheeler and Elliott (2008: 134) conclude that 'competent professional practice' involves:

- knowing what our methods are, and being able to discuss their merits and limitations
- knowing how to find new information from the literature (including electronic sources) that might help us with a particular client
- knowing how to access evidence to support our practice.

The discourse centred on the human mind is punctuated by certainties. Phrases that were earlier reserved for medical sciences, such as 'empirically supported' and 'clinically proven' treatments have become part of therapeutic reasoning.

This book is written in response to some of these changes and new requirements. It aims to demystify research and offers a step-by-step approach to conducting practice-based research, using current and relevant research as exemplars. The term 'demystifying' can have a sanitising ring to it. The aim is not to avoid the messiness and complexity of life. The book focuses rather on research – be it a 'private', everyday exploration or more systematically conducted studies – where the 'human factor' is taken into account. The research skills referred to in this book are linked to subjectivity and reflexivity. It will be argued that each piece of research will vary depending on the researcher who performs it. Reflexive awareness involves a deliberate attempt to position oneself as researcher in a linguistic, cultural, theoretical and personal context. Written with personal development as a guiding theme, the book encourages the reader to review, plan and find ways to take responsibility for her/his own learning and professional development in both research and clinical practice. The focus on personal development puts the researcher at the forefront; we are interested in how we position ourselves personally, theoretically and culturally in our research.

Public and private research

The term 'research' is used in a loose sense, akin to the definition suggested by Wengraf (2001: 4) in terms of 'getting a better understanding of the reality'. McLeod (1999: 8) asserts that all therapists by nature are practitioner researchers. Practice-based research is a broad concept; some of the key characteristics of practitioner research in therapy are:

- that the research question is triggered by personal experience and a 'need to know'
- that a goal is to produce knowledge that makes a positive difference to practice
- that an aim is to use reflexive awareness to access underlying meanings of the study.

Morris and Chenail (1994) offer a helpful distinction between private and public research. Private research involves 're-searching' interactions with our clients, on an everyday basis. Private research happens both in the moment, through our 'reflection-in-action' (Schön 1983) during sessions, and afterwards – through our case notes, supervision, peer support and continual professional development (CPT). Morris and Chenail (1994: 2) write:

> By *private research* we mean the type of inquiry which is done every day by reflecting practitioners in the course of their daily practice and they re-search their interactions both during conversations with clients and afterwards. The purpose of this research is to share the results of the inquiry with practitioners and clients. These studies are usually conducted informally and their results are used to make decisions in and about treatment.

The term 'public research' refers to a re-search process which is 'more formal in intent, structure, and execution', as Morris and Chenail (1994: 3) state:

> By *public research*, we mean those studies that are more formal in intent, structure, and execution. These are types of research that are presented at professional conferences and that are published in professional journals. The methods are clearly articulated, contexts of talk are analysed in intricate detail, and descriptions of clinical moments are rich and exhaustive.

Public research relies on private practice to progress, and vice versa. Clinical practitioners can, as Morris and Chenail (1994: 3) put it: 'private-ize' a whole range of methodologies and techniques to help them look 'beyond their private lenses'. It helps us, for instance, to trace our modalities to their underpinning, basic beliefs, and to challenge their consistency and more long-term implications.

Re-searching practice

Barkham et al. (2010) refer to practice-based research as a 'bottom-up' research. Practice-based research takes place on a grassroot level and involves practitioners and clients in a real-life setting. Practice-based inquiry involves revisiting and re-searching everyday events and as such often becomes both a 'personal journey of discovery' and a 'continual transformation process', as du Plock (2010: 122) reflects below:

> We get into difficulties, it seems to me, when we ... begin to see research as something different and separate from what we are already intimately involved in. ... We need to take more seriously the idea of research as a personal journey of discovery, or perhaps re-search, a continual transformation process rather than a discrete event.

We don't need to look far to find something to research. Practice-based research is, as suggested, an intrinsic part of our everyday life. Let us return to what can be described as 'private research', and to an example which highlights the complexity involved in 'assessing' situations and clients.

There is nothing so practical as a theory

Theory has, for many, got a dull ring to it. It tends to come across as something outside the practice. There is, as Lewin (1952) once addressed, 'nothing so practical as a theory'. Theories are the 'intellectual tools that guide practitioners' day-to-day and minute-to-minute clinical decision' (Stiles 2010: 91). Theories are 'ideas about the world conveyed in words, numbers, diagrams or other signs [which] offer distinct sets of assumptions and principles about the nature and sources of [for instance] psychological problems and about approaches and interventions to address them' (Stiles

2010: 91). Practice-based research encourages us to consider the choices we make with our clients in more detail. For instance, on what basis do we build our interpretations? How do we infer and reach conclusions regarding what may be true and false, right and wrong, in therapy? And do you test your theories in systematic ways? Or do you make a point of suspending any prior explanatory models when you are with your clients?

Our everyday life and practice is full of research. Sometimes the terms 'inductive' and 'deductive' reasoning are used to highlight whether the researcher starts his/her study with an open mind or with a plan to test a potential explanatory framework on something in the reality. This can be applied to clinical practice too. Inductive reasoning is typically characterised by 'unbiased' observations; it starts with an open mind and a deliberate attempt to suspend explanatory models or 'theories'. In contrast, deductive reasoning starts with a theory, or a well-formulated hypothesis, which is to be tested on selected sample groups.

Activity

As therapists, we are requested to choose between different theoretical orientations. How do we do that? On what basis do we arrive at knowledge and 'truths' within therapy? Read the case study below and consider the issues we have raised in the Reflection that follows. If possible, discuss how you might approach your work with Bill with a fellow student or colleague.

Case study

In spite of the door bell, there is a faint knock on the door.

'Hello, I've probably got the wrong house?' asks the man, as the therapist opens the door to let him in.

'Mr Gantt?'

The short, rather stocky man in his mid-30s nods in reply and continues talking while entering the room.

'Have any of your clients ever gone into the wrong building by mistake?', he chuckles.

'Have a seat ...'

'Anyway, yes, I am Mr Gantt. Call me Bill, by all means.'

Bill is wearing a suit and keeps flicking some invisible dust on his left thigh. He looks well attended to, with a crisp, white shirt and a tie. He sits with his legs wide apart. As he opens his mouth again to speak, tears begin to roll down his cheeks. He looks out of the window and speaks fast. Although he is crying, it is as if the tears have got nothing to do with him – as if they are not there.

'As I said on the phone, I've got a couple of issues at work that I'd like to discuss. There's been a promotion ... and, well, I'm also thinking about getting married. It's the second time around. My first wife attacked me with her high heeled shoes on our wedding night, so I'd rather avoid going down that route again!' He chuckles through his tears.

At this stage, the therapist decides to....

Reflection

What would *you* do at this stage? Some therapists start their first interview with an assessment questionnaire. Others aim for things to develop more 'organically'. Some may, for instance, argue that a relatively unstructured beginning allows valuable information about the client's way of relating to new situations to develop.

Would you, for instance, choose to let Bill develop his narrative further, uninterrupted – perhaps hoping to gain information about how Bill deals with new situations and people? Or would this be a good moment to change tack and bring out an assessment sheet or address some standard questions, perhaps with the view of considering mutual aims and objectives at as early a stage as possible? Or, is it likely that a different scenario would have emerged altogether had you been at the door to meet Bill? The way we approach our clients varies depending on our modality, personality and general approach to practice.

The psychoanalytic approach

A psychoanalytic therapist might, for instance, work with an object-relationships theory in mind. Hinshelwood (1997) addresses the 'point of maximum pain' in his assessment model. Where does the 'pain' or the problem really originate or belong? He suggests that we approach a client with a tripod in mind, where relationships to significant others have become a potential blueprint for subsequent relationships. Hinshelwood (1997: 157) writes:

Clinical material is best approached as pictures of relationships with objects. There are then three areas of object relationships which I try to bear in mind:

1. the current life situation
2. the infantile object relations, as described in the patient's history, or as hypothesised from what is known;
3. the relationship with the assessor which, to all intents and purposes, is the beginning of a transference.

The idea of 'transference' is an underlying principle for psychoanalytic practice. Transference was offered as a means of living through experiences, rather than simply thinking and talking about them. Freud (1940/1959: 41) considers the lived experience as a crucial aspect of the talking cure and asserts that 'the patient never forgets again what he has experienced in the form of transference'. Together with his colleague Breuer, Freud discovered that clients' anticipations of their therapists often coincided with their experiences from earlier relationships. Freud (1940/1959: 38) writes:

> The patient sees in his analyst the return – the reincarnation – of some important figure out of his childhood or past, and consequently transfers on to him feelings and reactions that undoubtedly applied to this model.

Transference contributes to the stereotype image of the silent, stern 'blank screen' analyst. The therapist's silence allows as much space as possible for transference. Transference 'comprises positive and affectionate as well as negative and hostile attitudes towards the analyst', writes Freud (1940/1959: 38). It is tempting, continues Freud (1940/1959: 39), to play into the role of a saviour, teacher and infallible helper, but we must 'shamefacedly admit' that it is often a question of the client's underlying 'aim of pleasing the analyst, of winning his applause and love' as means of repeating earlier patterns:

> However much the analyst may be tempted to act as teacher, model and ideal to other people and to make men into his own image, he should not forget that is not his task in the analytic relationship. ... He will only be repeating one of the mistakes of the parents, when they crushed their child's independence, and he will only be replacing one kind of dependency by another.

Deductive reasoning

The idea of transference and therapy as a space to relive, identify and challenge prior relationships (object-relations) reflects what, in research, is often referred to as a deductive reasoning; it becomes a theory to be tested and maybe refuted. Freud's deterministic model based on sexual drives is largely abandoned today; the term 'unconscious' is often used in a loose sense with reference to hitherto unexplored areas. However, psychoanalytic theory is increasingly incorporating neuroscientific theories on the 'unconscious', and these are guided by natural scientific and deductive reasoning. Neuro-psychoanalysis (Solms and Turnbull 2002) approaches the unconscious with reference to neurological processes, involving different kinds of cortices and memory functions. Kandel (2006: 281) asserts, for instance, that when we 'access' memories, core memories are 'elaborated upon and reconstructed, with subtractions, additions, elaborations and distortions':

> [R]ecalling a memory episodically – no matter how important the memory – is not like turning to a photograph in an album. Recall of memory is a creative process. What the brain stores is thought to be only a core memory. Upon recall, this core memory is then elaborated upon and reconstructed, with subtractions, additions, elaborations and distortions.

Schore (2003) specialises in our capacity to develop self-regulating emotions and assess how others feel about things. He focuses on how our affective and emotional development is influenced early on in life, and how it can be re-developed at later stages depending on circumstances. Schore (2003: 43) refers to the right brain as the 'locus of the emotional, corporeal, and the dynamic unconscious' and links its 'ongoing maturational potentials' to our 'attachment-influenced early organization'. He asserts that the early social environment influences the evolution of structures in the infant's brain. Schore suggests that the maturation of the orbitofrontal cortex is influenced by dyadic interactions of the attachment relationship. A neglected or impaired affect regulation can, argue Schore, be recovered; for instance, through psychotherapy. The relationship combines a *felt* experience with verbal conscious and intense reflective experiences, based on actual experiences of relating to others.

Humanistic theory

The humanistic (for instance, person-centred) therapist would meet Bill with 'therapist congruence' in mind and with an emphasis on what, in research terms, is called inductive reasoning. To be *in*congruent involves deliberately concealing aspects, for example, in a way which the psychoanalytically 'blank screen' therapist could be argued to do if she approaches Bill with an already formed hypothesis in mind. The therapeutic relationship taps into something which is already there, 'implicit, but unverbalised' in most clients. One of the overriding goals of therapy, suggests Rogers (1951: 150), is to work towards 'the dawning realization that the evidence upon which [the client] can base a value judgement is supplied by his [sic] own senses, his own experiences'. Not dissimilar from what Freud proposed earlier, Rogers (1951: 151) noted that many of his clients struggled with evaluating experiences. Rogers (1951: 149) concludes that 'it seems to be true that early in therapy the person is living largely by values he [sic] has introjected from his personal cultural environment'. Again, not unlike Freud, Rogers warned against the temptation to leap in and 'take over'. Rogers (1951: 151) writes:

> In therapy, in the initial phases, there appears to be a tendency for the locus of evaluation to lie outside the client. It is seen as a function of parents, of the culture, of friends, and of the counsellor. ... In client-centred therapy, however, one description of the counsellor's behaviour is that he consistently keeps the locus of evaluation with the client.

The person-centred therapist will, however, bring Bill's here and now to the forefront. Rogers (1951: 151) emphasises the importance of relating to clients in such a way that our responses, attitudes and phrases 'indicate that it is the client's evaluation of the situation which is accepted'. Rogers (1951, 1961, 1995) addressed certain core conditions for therapeutic change. Therapist 'unconditional positive regard' is a key core condition. The therapist is prepared to consider whether or not she is able to step into Bill's shoes and accept him unconditionally, without judgement, in order to give him space to explore his own 'locus of evaluation'. Unconditional positive regard is, asserts Rogers (1995: 116), about 'non-possessive caring'. Rogers writes:

> The therapist is willing for the client to be whatever immediate feeling is going on – confusion, resentment, fear, anger, courage, love, or pride. Such caring on the part of the therapist is nonpossessive. The therapist prizes the client in a total rather than a conditional way.

Rogers (1995: 14) compares congruence with being 'real':

> In place of the term 'realness' I have sometimes used the word 'congruence'. By this I mean *when my experiencing of this moment is present in my awareness and when my awareness is present in my communication*. (italics added)

Rogers believed in the impact of empathic understanding. A sense of being cared for by a genuine, honest person who aims to see things through the client's eyes with a 'no strings attached', unconditional interest became the bedrock of person-centred therapy.

Cognitive behavioural therapy

Cognitive behavioural therapy (CBT) includes a variety of approaches and therapeutic systems, some of the most well-known of which are cognitive therapy, rational emotive behaviour therapy and multimodal therapy. Cognitive behavioural therapy is based on collaborative effort to the extent that the therapeutic alliance is often compared with 'negotiation' (Gilbert and Leahy 2007: 92), although like the psychodynamic therapist who works with a hypothesis in mind, CBT is guided by deductive reasoning. Questions which a CBT therapist asks Bill may revolve around what logical errors could be involved in the way he perceives himself, his future and the world around him. Bill's therapist might use cognitive techniques such as examining the evidence and thought records to identify and change maladaptive cognitions. The therapist may also use behavioural methods to reverse ways of avoiding certain things through systematic exposure techniques. The term 'consciousness' is used in CBT as a state where rational decisions can be said to be made with full awareness. 'Automatic' thoughts are often used to describe an opposite form of making decisions. These refer to what Beck called 'private cognitions'. Much of Bill's cognitions could be described as automatic thoughts. They are shaped by his prior experiences and have become core beliefs or schemas which create templates for the way he processes information in the present. CBT refers to a Socratic method which encourages clients to contribute by asking questions of themselves: 'How do I really know that all people are dangerous? What is the logic in that? Could they seem threatening because they are in a bad mood or because I have approached them in a reserved, maybe defensive, way?', and so on. Homework is likely to become a part of Bill's therapeutic process if he undertakes CBT. He and his therapist will agree on tasks which Bill can do in between sessions to explore his automatic thoughts in terms of facts.

Beck et al. (1987: 50, 54) assert that 'therapeutic interaction is based on trust, rapport and collaboration' and they view it as a 'vehicle to facilitate a common effort in carrying out specific goals'. As Beck et al. (1987) contend, cognitive approaches often seem deceptively easy. Both Rogers' core conditions and Freud's idea of transference are noted in his approach to the 'therapeutic alliance'. Warmth, assert Beck et al. (1987: 46), is essential to establish a therapeutic relationship, although 'it is crucial to bear in mind that the patient's response is his [sic] perception of warmth rather than the actual degree of warmth expressed by the therapists'. Beck et al. also emphasise genuineness and empathy: the therapist must be able 'to experience life the way the patient does' at the same time as being 'careful not to project his [sic] own attitude or expectations onto the patient'. This empathic understanding will, continue Beck et al. (1987: 48), be balanced with 'objective checking of the patient's introspection against other sources of information', such as 'testing the logic involved in the patient's inferences and conclusions'. However, CBT emphasises overall the collaborative problem-solving approach which Beck et al. referred to above.

Growing rabbit ears

Yalom (2002: 52) writes about 'growing rabbit ears' right from the start to pick up on the often subtle, but 'informative idiosyncratic responses' brought by his clients to same-situation scenarios. He describes, for instance, how walking down to his office along a winding path from his house has helped him 'accumulate much comparison data':

> You must grow rabbit ears. The everyday events of each therapy session are rich with data: consider how your patients greet you, take a seat ... [T]he patient's idiosyncratic response is ... a *via regia*, permitting you to understand the patient's inner world. (Yalom 2002: 52)

Yalom's observations illustrate an attempt to be guided by each client's unique responses, and to approach meaning-making processes with as open a mind as possible. In research terms, this is often referred to as 'inductive' reasoning. Yalom (2002: 52) continues:

> My office is in a separate cottage about a hundred feet down a winding garden path, I have over the years accumulated much comparison data. Most patients comment about the garden ... but some do not. One man never failed to make some negative comment: the mud on the path, the need for guardrails in the rain ... [When] the latch on my screen door was broken, preventing the door from closing

snugly, my patients responded in a number of ways. One patient invariably spent much time fiddling with it and each week apologised for it as though she had broken it. Many ignored it, while others never failed to point out the defect and suggest I should get it fixed.

A therapist informed by object-relations theory might, for instance, attempt some deductive reasoning to make sense of why the lady 'fiddles' apologetically with Yalom's door and hypothesise that she is transferring some of her earlier relationship experiences on to the therapeutic relationship. If this theory is refuted by another explanation, the therapist may consider eliminating it from the search. Humanistic therapists, like Yalom himself, would typically approach their clients for the first time with an open mind and put explanatory frameworks to the side. Humanistic psychology developed during the 1950s in direct opposition to the idea of therapy as a form of 'excavation'. Yalom (1980: 10) writes:

> To Freud, exploration always meant excavation. ... Deepest conflict meant earliest conflict. ... There is no compelling reason to assume that 'fundamental' (that is, important, basic) and 'first' (that is, chronologically first) are identical. To explore deeply from an existential perspective does not mean that one explore the past; rather it means that one brushes away everyday concerns and thinks deeply about one's existential situation.

Inductive reasoning is favoured where a sense of explanation grows in the context of each individual client. The therapeutic frame can still be used as a 'base line', as Yalom (2002: 157) puts it, to learn something about the variations and differences between clients and their reactions:

> I develop baseline expectations because all my patients encounter the same person (assuming I am reasonably stable), receive the same directions to my office, enter the same room with the same furnishing.

Activity

Every session is a piece of research

McLeod (1994, cited by du Plock 2010: 122) reminds us about how we are constantly engaged in 'practice research', as part of our daily clinical work:

> A counselling session with a client can be seen as a piece of research, a piecing together of information and understandings, followed by testing the validity of conclusions and actions based on shared knowing.

- Try to think about a session with a client as a piece of research. Consider how you piece together information and understandings, followed by testing the validity of conclusions and actions based on shared knowing.

How open can a mind be?

The prospect of suspending explanatory models in favour of *unbiased* observations, as in the case of Yalom's walks towards his private practice at the end of the garden, assumes that prior knowledge and expectations actually *can* be separated from what we see. An often-addressed problem with 'inductive' reasoning is, for example, as Warburton (2004) asserts, that our knowledge and our expectation affect what we see. Warburton (2004: 112) writes:

> the simple view assumes that our knowledge and expectations do not affect our observations. [However] seeing something isn't just having an image on your retina. ... Our knowledge and our expectations of what we are likely to see affect what we actually do see.

The therapist as a person

A particularly important aspect in psychotherapy is to challenge our pre-understanding, with a focus on our emotional, affective responses and expectations. Countertransference was initially a concept designed to understand what the therapist felt in relation to the client's transference. It was regarded as something that always 'came', or was projected, from the client. Racker (2001) asserts that psychotherapy always involved a fusion between the past and the present for *both* therapists and clients, and he refers to different types of countertransference, for instance, Concordant and Complementary countertransference. At times, reactions in the therapist will stem from the client's transference and projection towards the therapist. It is important, argues Racker, to acknowledge how some issues tap into the therapist's own history. Clarkson (1995: 9) suggests that therapists need to listen to their reactions in terms of 'reactive' and 'proactive' countertransference.

- *Reactive countertransference* describes the psychotherapist's feelings which are elicited by or induced by the patient.
- *Proactive countertransference* refers to feelings, atmospheres, projections, etc. which can be said to have been introduced by the psychotherapist him/herself.

What if, for instance, one of the clients 'fiddling' with Yalom's door triggers some of Yalom's own old memories? What if the person is an overweight, middle-aged woman? The terms transference and countertransference helps us to conceptualise the impact that prior relationships can have on the way we experience people later on.

Although Yalom works within an existential framework, he stresses that countertransference and transference can be useful 'tools' (i.e. theory) for conceptualising how emotional pre-understandings impact our observations. In one of his case studies, Yalom (1991: 87) captures some of the strong feelings involved for him as a therapist when he meets Betty, a client with weight issues:

> The day that Betty entered my office, the instant I saw her steering her ponderous two-hundred-and-fifty frame towards [me], I knew that a great trial of countertransference was in store for me. I have always been repelled by fat women. I find them disgusting: their sidewise waddle, their absence of body contour ... everything obscured in an avalanche of flesh. ... How dare they impose that body on the rest of us? The origins of these sorry feelings? [W]ere an explanation demanded of me, I ... would point to the family of fat, controlling women, including – featuring – my mother, who peopled my early life.

Yalom (1991: 87) concludes that knowledge about the therapist's emotive responses to their clients is an essential aspect of 'the inexhaustible curriculum of self improvement':

> The world's finest tennis players train five hours a day ... the ballerina [endlessly aspires] to consummate balance, the priest forever examines his conscious .... For psychotherapists that realm, that inexhaustible curriculum of self improvement from which he never graduates, is referred to in the trade as countertransference. Where transference refers to feelings that the patient erroneously attaches ('transfers') to the therapists but that in fact originated out of earlier relationships, countertransference is the reverse – similar irrational feelings that the therapist has towards the patient.

Self-awareness is, for a therapist, the equivalence of 'consummating balance' for a ballerina; it is, as Yalom (2002) suggests, a significant part of the therapist's 'inexhaustible curriculum of self improvement'. This kind of self-awareness is, however, often a neglected area in research. Emotional responses are something which traditionally have been regarded as obstacles rather than as something which informs and enriches the inquiry.

Activity

Time travelling

Real-world research is based on the world that we live in. The world we live in involves the past, present and our future – whether we are clients, therapists, research participants or researchers. This writing exercise is about one of the many cornerstones of your world and reality. In this activity, you are encouraged to write for ten minutes without stopping. As Winter et al. (1999: 11) describe:

> Uninterrupted writing [means] to get down and write. If you cannot think of the next word, then repeat the one you are writing until the one you need occurs to you. Don't spend time wondering what to write next.

Continue writing from the sentence below for five minutes without stopping!

'I remember it was a school day, maybe a Tuesday or a Wednesday. I was sitting on my bed, looking for a sock, thinking that ...'
   When you have finished:

- Trace how you are feeling right now.
- What came up for you?
- How old was the person you wrote about? What happened to that person, at that time?

When I have undertaken this exercise with clients, some clients have expressed surprise over the amount of detail that comes out in the writing, such as smells, sounds and other vivid memories linked to time and place. Others comment sometimes on how little comes out. For instance, in one writing group, a member described feeling almost paralysed, unable to write a single word. He was later able to reflect over how this actually coincided with his feelings both at home and in school at this particular time. Many describe how strong feelings can return in their writing, such as sadness, helplessness and loneliness – or, indeed, in some cases, excitement. One person remembered the day his mother was being hospitalised and memories of trying to make sense of all this when he came to school flooded back. This triggered a discussion about how many in the group where 'wounded healers', who could recall a sense of leading a double-life as children, with a messy household and an urge to fit in and be a 'normal' child at school. Often, the writers are surprised afterwards to recognise that the age wasn't specified in the exercise, and that the feeling they had about being asked to write about themselves with a special age in mind was linked to their own way of prioritising events. In one writing group, a member said afterwards that she found it easy to write: 'It was the grey sock that did it for me' she said. Only afterwards did she recognise that this was in response to what had come up for her, rather than being specifically addressed in the question.

Recommended reading

McLeod, J. (2013) *An Introduction to Research in Counselling and Psychotherapy.* London: Sage.

McLeod gives an excellent overview of the different stages and angles to counselling research.

TWO Personal development

The purpose with personal development in training is to increase awareness of how practitioners' own personality, behaviour and cultural values can impact decision makings and relationships at work. This level of self-awareness is often neglected in research. This chapter places the researcher at the forefront and explores how prior personal and professional experiences are being integrated in both practice and research.

- Frameworks for understanding
- Reflective research
- Critical reflection
- Self-knowledge
- Methodological approach
- Qualitative and quantitative research
- Phenomenology
- Mixed methods

The concept personal development is commonly used on training and staff development programmes to explore the 'engine that drives us'. It revolves around the way we understand and integrate personal and professional experiences in our practice. In this chapter, we will approach systematic or 'public' research without losing sight of the researcher as a person.

Reflective research

In the last chapter, we looked at how du Plock (2010: 122) addressed practice-based research as a means of 're-searching' what we are already involved in, with the view to embracing 'continual transformation'. Looking at something familiar through a new lens is at the root of practice-based and work-based research; framings and frame reflections are key components in reflective practice, as Costley et al. (2010: 160) assert:

[A]n important characteristic of work based research [is] its capacity to make explicit knowledge that is often taken for granted or tacit. ... As a work based researcher, you have at your disposal an immensely valuable resource – your own experience of the workplace. However, in order to turn this experience into knowledge ... it will be necessary to create knowledge through the 'transformation of experience'.

The above-mentioned 'transformation of experience' involves a critical exploration of the way we work – as individuals and in our agency or organisation. This process involves, as Doncaster (2000: 155) describes:

learning to critically reflect on past experience, to organise learning into discrete areas and argue a case for why such learning is [academically] worthy. ... The teasing out, organising and grouping of experiential learning is in itself a learning process – [researchers] learn how to reflect on their experience, how to identify their own patterns of learning, and to [work] decisions on the basis of this self-knowledge.

If we, for instance, decide to evaluate an agency in which we have worked for many years, say a school-based therapy service, we need to communicate our enthusiasm and reasons for involvement – i.e. describe why we are interested in this in the first place – but we also need to adopt a critical 'creative indifference'. Exploring something from as many different and new perspectives as possible invariably involves stages where we will feel disorientated and deskilled. Familiar frameworks suddenly become skewed and alien as part of our process of adopting new and potentially different angles to our work. An example which has stayed in my mind regarding eye-opening practice-based research is when a friend undertook a study about narratives in therapy. She was 'appalled', she wrote, to recognise how 'active' she was in the sessions. Having to scrutinise her own practice caused her to recognise just how influential her own voice was in session narratives. The study triggered her to reconsider her image of herself as a therapist altogether; she had a feeling of 'putting words' into her clients' mouth:

We're at a stage of our research when we feel appalled by our own practice. My colleague, who recorded my sessions, allowed me to read the transcripts, and I was appalled to learn about how much I actually speak in my sessions. I've always pictured myself as a bit of a nodding listener, with an occasional well-chosen intervention. Seeing the transcripts gave me a totally new insight into how the clients' narratives take shape; I had naively thought they somehow developed in isolation from me. My research has prompted me to think long and hard on how I interact with my clients. It has shaken me to the core. (Anonymous)

Researchers will need to put themselves 'in the shoes of other actors [and show] the complementary ability to consider how their own frames may contribute to the problematic situations', as Schön (1983: 187) puts it. Costley et al. (2010: 120) refer to reflective practice 'as an invaluable approach, to think about theory building and conceptual frameworks' in practice-based research. Costley et al. (2010: 117–18) continue:

> [T]he notion of the reflective practitioner ... provides a conceptual framework within [which] the complexities, tensions and contradictions of work can be explored, and at the same time a reference point against [which] the intrinsic value and practice can be judged. [It] opens up the possibility of exploring practice from a variety of perspectives. ... For the work based researcher [reflective practice] is a powerful tool for uncovering otherwise hidden process, decision paths and power relations in the work place. It helps the researcher move beyond mere description to analysis.

Schön (1983: 310) suggests that when 'a practitioner becomes aware of his [sic] frames, he also becomes aware of the possibility of alternative ways of framing the reality of his practice. He takes notes of the values and norms to which he has given priority, and those he has given less importance, or left out of account altogether.'

New perspectives on our practice – locating ourselves in the greater world

'We all need to place ourselves within the context of the greater world', writes Marie Adams (2012: 126ff) in her research about the personal lives of therapists. She refers to research as a means not only of learning about the world around us, but also of 'mak[ing] sense of who we are':

> We all need to place ourselves within the context of the greater world to give us significance, perhaps, and certainly a sense of place. We need to create a story for ourselves and make sense of who we are. I used to scribble in my notebook: Marie Adams, Monstrose Street, Winnipeg, Manitoba, Canada, North America, the World, the Universe. I feel both a million miles, and yet not so far away from that little girl writing out her address across the front of her exercise books, unconsciously working hard to place herself in context. Research, I believe, is often simply the grown up version of that same pre-occupation. (Adams 2012: 126)

Marie's research is another illustrative example of practice-based research which takes place in our everyday practice, carried out by the practitioners themselves. This research revolves around the therapists' own boundaries and coping mechanisms:

> My research involved interviewing forty therapists across three countries and ten therapists in each of four major traditions: psychoanalytic, integrative, humanistic and cognitive behavioural. I wanted to know how they believed their personal lives affected their work with clients/patients and how other therapists had experienced themselves as professionals working through hard times. If faced with the same circumstances again, would they conduct themselves differently? Would they continue working? (Adams 2012: 126)

Practice-based research often starts with a critical incident which has affected us or triggered some more systematic investigations. An important aspect of practice-based research is, as suggested, the emphasis on personal development, and to 'own' the research interest, rather than conceal it, or maybe use research participants to address it. Underneath Marie's interest were some very personal questions:

> My research began after struggling through a particularly difficult period of five months, following a professional complaint. ... In my case, I was fortunate enough that the complaint was dropped, but none the less, if trauma can be evoked from what we imagine might happen, rather than what actually takes place, I was certainly affected ... I had lived in a state of almost overwhelming anxiety and fear that the career I had worked so hard for might be yanked from underneath me, and linked with that, of course, would be profound shame when the news became public. ... I did spend some time in a dark tunnel. ... From this apparently unfortunate beginning the seed of my research was planted, helping me to give meaning to my experience and place myself within the context of a greater therapeutic community. ... When I eventually emerged, I felt both grateful and overwhelmed by the number of 'stories' I was told by other therapists who had faced traumatic events while working. The stories included life-threatening illnesses, bereavement and professional crisis, among them redundancy and professional complaints. (Adams 2012: 127)

Marie Adams wanted to learn more about other therapists' experiences of integrating personal issues into their professional lives, and this interest guided her towards a qualitative approach. It is important to consider in research the differences between qualitative and quantitative approaches. The choices of theoretical frameworks will affect the outcome of the study.

Qualitative research is, as Pistrang and Barker (2010: 67) assert, 'particularly valuable for investigating the personal meanings that people attach to their experiences'. Pistrang and Barker (2010: 67) distinguish between 'thematic' analysis and 'language-focused' approaches within the qualitative framework. Phenomenology, narrative analysis and content analysis are some alternatives within the thematic approach. One way of looking for and capturing meaning-making processes is by identifying themes in their stories. Interpretive Phenomenological Analysis (IPA) is 'a particularly user-friendly version' (Pistrang and Barker 2010: 75) among phenomenological approaches. IPA does not rely on random sampling in the way that, for instance, evidence-based research proposes (as we shall see later). The sample can be 'purposive, because you purposively set out to recruit only those who share the experience being investigated', concludes Langridge (2007: 58). The aim is to 'gather detailed information about the experience of a fairly specific group on a fairly specific topic', continues Langridge (2007: 110), as he reflects over the researcher's approach to his/her research participants:

> The researcher constructs an interview schedule consisting of a number of open-ended questions on the topic being investigated. These might include questions asking the participant to describe and reflect on different aspects of

their experience, such as the impact on their sense of self, family and friends and with their methods of coping. Interviews are normally tape-recorded and then transcribed verbatim. (Langridge 2007: 110)

Qualitative research is often 'concerned with making sense of the participant's world', and thematic analysis approaches meaning-making processes and subjective experiences as 'major themes', writes Langridge (2007: 111):

> Thematic analysis is the principle analytical approach used with IPA. Essentially, the analyst is concerned with making sense of the participant's world and, therefore, spends a considerable amount of time working through the transcripts (and listening to the tape) in order to identify the major themes.

Phenomenology is a complex and rich approach, and an area to which we will return. On a very simple level, we can say that using a single case as the starting point, the researcher adopting IPA usually proceeds through the following stages. Langridge (2007: 111) continues:

> **Stage 1:** read and re-read, adding comments into the left-hand margin about the meaning of particular sections. ... Comments may be summaries, associations or the aim is simply to state what is going on in the text ...

> **Stage 2:** emerging themes are noted in the right-hand margin. Initial notes are transformed into more meaningful statements, reflecting a broader level of meaning in a particular section of the text ...

> **Stage 3:** themes are listed separately on paper. ... The analyst now attempts to identify common links between themes and to reorder them in a more analytical or theoretical way. Some themes will cluster together. ... Some will appear to be more subordinate themes ...

> **Stage 4:** the analyst now produces a table of themes in a coherent order ... appropriately named [and] linked to the originating text.

Once this is done, the researcher can either begin from scratch with the next transcribed interview, or adopt the table of themes from the previous analysis as a guide and work her way through the interviews in that way. Adams (2012: 126ff) included an unusually large sample group, given the time-consuming nature of the thematic analysis. She interviewed, as mentioned earlier, forty therapists:

> One of the most significant results from my research was the amount of depression experienced by therapists during their period of working. Of the forty therapists interviewed, more than half (24) admitted they had suffered depression in the course of their working lives. Of these, sixteen psychotherapists said their experience was episodic, while the remaining eight described themselves as suffering 'chronic' depression. Breaking this down even further, 13 therapists in this group suffered a form of abandonment as children, including parental

death, an alcoholic parent and neglect. Only three therapists who named aban-
donment of some kind in their childhood did not experience depression ...

While some therapists described their depression as completely debilitating at
times, those who described their experience as 'chronic', tended to live with it
and function regardless, often through the support of therapy and sometimes in
conjunction with medication. One therapist, though, admitted that therapy did
not work for her; she knew all the 'tricks', and she relied on drugs to help her
through the difficult periods.

As suggested earlier, this kind of research will almost invariably throw new
light on previously shaded areas – both with regard to our own and other
people's clinical practice. Marie (Adams 2012: 129) continues:

In learning about [other therapists] I thought, I might learn something to my
benefit, and by extension, so might others. Perhaps what I really wanted was
reassurance, to know that I wasn't alone in my experience ...

What I hadn't planned on was to what an extent I would learn, and to what
degree it would affect me in my work as a therapist. Through considering how
other psychotherapists had coped, I was forced to look at my own feelings of
omnipotence, my vulnerability to shame, the impossibility of perfection and that
reassuring certainty that I belong to a community – the world, the universe.

Integrating personal experiences in professional development

The purpose of personal development training is, as Spencer (2006: 109)
puts it, to help students and staff 'increase their awareness of how their
personality, behaviour, personal and cultural beliefs might impact on, and
influence, their clients'. Personal development includes linking past with
present, and vice versa. Neuhaus (2011: 224) defines personal development in terms of a process where you are encouraged to consider how you
'react as a person with emotions, thoughts and behaviour both inside and
outside [your work]'. This includes, as Neuhaus (2011: 224) puts it, 'attending one's personal history (e.g. life span development, identity development and family relationships) that may have a significant influence on the
ways in which [we] react'.

Stephen Adams-Langley shares the background to his research into school-
based therapy below. He works at a national children's charity that provides
counselling in schools. Stephen's research highlights how the personal can be
integrated in both practice and research, and addresses questions about how
to handle an 'insider' perspective, which may potentially lead to a biased
outlook. Stephen has chosen a so-called grounded theory for his research,
which combines inductive and deductive reasoning – i.e. it attempts to make
unbiased observations as well as test a theory. We will return to this when
we explore methodology and reflexivity in more detail. At this point,

Stephen's musing over his research interest acts as an example of what, in personal development terms, is called 'integrating personal experiences in the professional development'.

Case study

Stephen formulates his research question as:

'The Place2Be in the Inner City: How Can a Voluntary Sector Mental Health Service Have an Impact on Children's Mental Health and the School Environment?'

Stephen (Adams-Langley 2011: 135) concludes that he aims 'to bring alive the voices and qualitative experience of the key players in the service, and rather than present *evidence-based practice*, present the narrative of *practice-based evidence*, through qualitative inquiry and field-based exploration and explanation'.

He reflects over his research interest on different levels. He introduces his own organisation, and reflects over school-based counselling in the context of other, ongoing research as well as his own personal investment.

Stephen's research resulted in a doctorate dissertation. The experience involved learning on different levels. Below are some extracts from his reflections regarding the choice of research subject.

General background for the research

A child's formative years has a huge impact on their development and long term prospects. It is estimated that more than one million children in the United Kingdom under the age of fifteen have a diagnosable mental health problem, but a high proportion of these children do not receive a mental health intervention. A recent analysis of a large scale longitudinal study (Kim-Cohen, Caspi, Moffitt, Harrington and Milne, 2003), indicated that seventy-five per cent of those who met criteria for one of the seventeen mental disorders at twenty-six years of age had a disorder diagnosed by the age of eighteen, fifty-seven per cent by the age of fifteen. A third of those treated for depression at the age of twenty-six, had diagnosable mood symptoms in childhood. (Adams-Langley 2011: 5–6)

Specific reference to Place2Be

The Place2Be is a charity and voluntary organisation that was established in 1994, to improve the emotional well-being of children, their families, teachers and the school community. The Place2Be primarily works in primary schools, but over the past five years has established a school based mental health programme in one hundred and seventy-two primary schools, and piloted a successful model of therapeutic support to fourteen secondary schools for pupils in years seven and eight (pupils aged eleven to thirteen), to support children with transition and emotional and psychological difficulties. (Adams-Langley 2011: 56)

Stephen (Adams-Langley 2011: 20, 14) also places his interest and motivation in the context of personal experiences and *positions the research in the context of both personal and professional learning*:

> On a professional level, I hope to reveal the case for early intervention through counselling in schools, with a particular emphasis on 'hard to reach' children, with multiple risk factors living in the inner city. A focus of this doctorate will be to consider the 'hard to reach' child living in the inner city, who may be experiencing several risk factors due to poverty and deprivation. Further to this, there is a tentative hypothesis that the provision of an accessible school-based intervention may encourage resilience in the child, and emotional support for children living in some of the most challenging circumstances in London. Although I have managed several Place2Be services in Nottingham, Medway and Cardiff, as well as Enfield, Lambeth and Camden, where there are many children who have had similar life circumstances, I will concentrate this study in areas in the inner city in London where I have managed the Place2Be programmes for fourteen years. I hope to reveal the impact on children, the adults who support them, and the school community...

On a *personal level*, Stephen (Adams-Langley 2011: 20, 14) relates to his research interest as follows:

> It is obviously no coincidence that I have developed the role as the Child Protection and Safe Guarding Officer in the Place2Be charity in the past fourteen years, and worked to promote child mental health, and the need to foster emotional resilience in children. ... My personal motivation is inevitably based on my experiences as a child and adolescent. If I consider my own risk factors, I was a child from a highly volatile family structure with early and enduring experiences of parental rejection and ambivalence. I have written about my experience as a child and experiencing Munchhausen by proxy ... with frequent hospitalisations and poor attendance at school leading to isolation, school refusal and academic failure. ... Masten et al. (1990) describe resilience as 'the process of or opportunity for successful adaptation despite difficult or threatening circumstances'. Despite my difficult circumstances, I did possess relatively high self-esteem, and a belief that I could endure into adult life, where I would have autonomy, flexibility and freedom. .... Sedgwick (1994) writes of the 'wounded helper' and the 'wounded physician' in Jungian therapy, and my brief description of some aspects of my own childhood and experience at school will be illuminated in this research into school based mental health for children. ... I hope ... that the 'voices' and perception of the key players are revealed through qualitative research employing grounded theory, case studies and a co-operative inquiry.

Activity

Personal development in research

Discuss how professional and personal experiences are being reflected upon by Stephen in his research. Can you apply the same approach as part of your own research interest? How would you describe your professional *and* personal investment in your research? Discuss, if possible, in pairs. Some prompts might be:

- Where do you work? What do you do?
- What knowledge, skills and personal qualities have you developed so far? What do you feel most proud of?
- What do you feel excited or passionate about?
- What values/beliefs/worldview have you embraced? How would you, for instance, describe your therapeutic modality?
- List three or four areas or topics which you could consider researching. Maybe they are linked to a personal experience, a general need to know or represent a means to enhance work, either your own or someone else's practice.

Quantitative or qualitative research?

We have already referred to how quantitative studies tend to build on deductive reasoning, and will in this sense involve tests with specific variables and well-defined hypotheses. The 'hypothesis or measurable statement' that can be deduced from a theory, will, as Moule and Hek (2011: 63) put it, 'be tested' to either support the prediction and confirm the theory or not.

According to Giacomini (2001), quantitative research tends to 'answer questions such as whether? (e.g. whether an intervention did more good than harm?), or how much? (e.g. how strongly does a risk factor predispose to a disease?).'

Giacomini (2001: 2) illustrates the difference using a traffic light metaphor. Quantitative research can measure real things, such as the number of cars which stop for a red light. Qualitative research can help us understand more about the drivers' perception and experience of the traffic lights, and can explore why drivers behave in the way they do.

> If we want to cross the street, the quantitative traffic study allows us to estimate the likelihood of getting run over, and on this basis, we can take an informed chance. However, the implied 'law' that traffic light colour makes cars go and stop would be useless if we want to reform drivers or simply understand them. The qualitative study gives more insight into why people do what they do.

In the case of quantitative research, a hypothesis is formulated about, for instance, whether a green light causes cars to drive. Giacomini (2001: 3) continues:

Quantitative researcher might hypothesise that red lights make cars stop, whereas green ones make them go. Researchers could randomly expose cars to red and green lights and record stopping and going responses. ... The study might disprove the hypothesis that the green light has less effect than the red light on stopping and going; it might estimate the likelihood of a car running a red light or sitting through a green one.

Activity

Consider what kind of survey you would undertake using the traffic lights? What would you be curious to know more about regarding the drivers' behaviours? What kinds of questions would you like to ask?

An important starting point in systematic quantitative research is to consider how different kinds of questions will produce different kinds of data. For instance, to what extent do the questions posed capture nominal, ordinal, interval or ratio data.

- The 'nominal' concept refers to data with named rather than arithmetic values, such as male/female or train/car.
- Ordinal categories reflect different kinds of order and relationships, expressing them by degree, such as using categories like 'agree' versus 'disagree' (we shall read more about this in the next chapter).
- Interval categories can also be ranked in different kinds of order, but with equal intervals between the categories. An example of an interval scaling is temperature.
- Ratio categories or data have a zero point, just like the interval scales, but while 30°C cannot be said to be twice as hot as 15 degrees, the ratio categories can claim this kind of 'double as' or 'half as' relationship. Examples of ratio categories are income or age.

Reflection

What kind of category would your data fall within?

Depending on what the categories are measuring, different forms of descriptive statistics can be chosen to analyse and present the data. There are different forms of frequency tables to present the data, for instance, a pie chart can be used to illustrate the relative proportions of a certain aspect, and a bar chart can be used to compare data across categories.

An important aim in quantitative research is usually, as Whittaker (2009: 101) addresses, 'to report a typical or average value'. The 'mean' is a common term in research. It refers to the numerical value we get 'by adding up the value of all of the responses and dividing the total by the number of responses received' (Whittaker 2009: 101). The 'mean' is only relevant on categories which can be counted, such as data in interval and ratio scales. The 'median' is a useful measuring term for describing ordinal data. We can, for instance, rank an agreement on a scale from lowest to highest, for example from strongly disagree to strongly agree, and aim for a median in terms of a mid-point in the set of ranked orders. If, on the other hand, we would like to compare the amount of cars which stopped or did not stop for a red light in the example of the traffic lights mentioned above, then 'mode' is a useful type of average. Mode captures the category with the highest frequency, and can be used for nominal as well as numerical data, i.e. in all four categories of data mentioned above.

Sampling techniques are particularly significant to consider in quantitative research. As Sanders and Wilkins (2010) assert, an overriding aim in quantitative research is to keep the researcher's personal interest out of the equation. It is particularly important to avoid sampling biases. A sample reflects a part of the target population from which information is collected – for instance, cars which pass through the traffic lights during, say, Mondays and Saturdays. The sampling trustworthiness ranges from random sampling to convenience sampling with a sampling frame of, for instance, the drivers who are easiest to approach – the latter sampling is 'the weakest sampling technique because bias may be introduced from the sample' (Moule and Hek 2011: 95).

While quantitative research can be extremely useful in estimating the likelihood of getting run over before crossing the road, for example, a qualitative study will provide more insight into why people do what they do:

> Qualitative reports offer access and insight into particular social settings, activities, or experiences. In contrast to quantitative approaches, qualitative research neither presumes that predetermined variables or causal relationships exist nor tries to find them. (Giacomini 2001: 3)

Qualitative research approaches the traffic behaviour as a social phenomenon. Giacomini (2001: 3) continues:

> Qualitative researchers would approach traffic behaviour as a symbolically mediated social phenomenon. At the outset, the researchers would assume they know little about people's reasons for doing what they do or what their actions mean. Researchers would ask, 'what do these lights mean to drivers, and why do they respond the way they do?' They might interview drivers, read traffic law, observe behaviour at traffic lights, and try driving. On the basis of various information sources, they would develop a theory of driving behaviour and report that green means 'go' and red means 'stop' (or to some, red means 'go if you can get away with it'). The open ended research question allows the researchers to discover the yellow light and its role.

Moule and Hek (2011: 58) assert that an inductive approach in research 'encapsulates the philosophy that people are fundamentally different to things':

> Inductive reasoning moves from the general to the particular ... it usually starts off with a set of observations. From this very early stage the researcher would plan to document the information very carefully. This inductive approach in research encapsulates the philosophy that people are fundamentally different to things, and should be valued as individuals. As patterns of behaviour or interactions develop, the researchers seek to make sense of them from the individual's perspective.

Choosing the 'right' methodological approach

Many practice-based researchers find that they gravitate towards research which is congruent with their clinical modality. Stephen Adams-Langley reflects over how his existential outlook marries well with his choice, grounded theory.

> As an existential humanistic psychotherapist, I value the phenomenological method to elicit subject meaning and experience, and grounded theory is a qualitative methodology aligned to this world view. (Adams-Langley 2011: 28)

Anne refers, for instance, to her methodological approach with reference to her psychoanalytic practice:

> Regarding the research methodology, as a psychoanalytic psychotherapist conducting a small scale qualitative inquiry, I knew that I wanted my research to reflect the mind-set I inhabit in my professional life and work, desiring that the research sought to inquire beneath the words spoken in an interview, looking at what was unspoken as well as spoken in a bid to make meaning out of each participant's story. (Anne)

These two options both fall within the category of qualitative research. As Beverley reflects below, qualitative research tends to marry well with the open approach of psychotherapy. But there are sometimes equally valid reasons to research within a quantitative framework. Beverley writes:

> In psychotherapy, we focus on attending to individuals' voices and their subjective experiences. We are also aware of the impossibility of taking a neutral stance. ... This would incline me more towards qualitative methods, such as grounded theory, which value the meaning which can be generated from in-depth interviews with a small number of participants, while taking into account the social constructionist view that meaning is made through interaction with each other and with the social world. ... However, with qualitative research, sample sizes are often very small. We wanted to create as big a body of evidence as possible for this under-researched area to be taken seriously. I had no experience of quantitative forms of research and I had my own prejudices.

As will be shown in the following chapter, Beverley found that a mixed-methods approach captured both her interests. Mixed methods are used for various reasons. Apart from the option of combining an interest in large sample populations with a focus on unique meaning-making processes, mixed methods are sometimes used in underdeveloped research areas where traditional approaches provide unsatisfactory explanatory frameworks. Western philosophy and science have developed with a focus on white, middle-class males. As we shall see later in this book, researchers with an interest in cross-cultural or transgender-related aspects tend to find that traditional methods provide insufficient support for their studies; an argument is being raised for the need for new combinations and variations of explanatory frameworks to develop, and the argument for mixed methods is being raised in this debate. On a more traditional basis, arguments are being put forward for mixed methods on the grounds that it helps to triangulate and validate methods. If the qualitative research is supported by a quantitative exploration, or vice versa, the researchers can argue that their data has been tested from different angles.

As with the other methodological approaches, the choice is also often linked to the researcher's previous experiences and regular clinical practice. Practice-based research expects the researcher to be as reflective and transparent as possible with regard to these choices. Another example of this kind of transparency is offered in the case study below, where Alan Priest reflects over his choice to work with both quantitative and qualitative methodologies.

Case study

Mixed methods research has been defined as 'the collection or analysis of both quantitative and qualitative data in a single study in which the data are collected concurrently or sequentially, are given a priority, and involve the integration of the data at one or more stages in the process of research'. ... In selecting a mixed methods approach my intention was, as some suggest ... to approach the qualitative and quantitative elements as complementary parts of my attempt to meet the aims of my study, incorporating an element of triangulation to enhance its usefulness and reliability. ... I trained and worked originally as a chemist. Here, the combination of qualitative and quantitative approaches to analysis was entirely normal and natural. Admittedly, in the laboratory environment, both methods are utilised within the same overall scientific paradigm but even so, I remain convinced that combining different approaches in pursuit of certain research problems is entirely appropriate. ... I therefore invite you the reader to share in my paradigm; I believe the strength of my approach lies is its ability to illuminate 'what happened (for the client) when ...' and 'how often this happened', linking both of these categories of knowing, respectively, to subjective perception and quantification of effect. (Priest 2013: 102–3)

Activity

Ask yourself the following questions:

- How do you work?
- On what basis do you generate knowledge in your practice?
- How does this relate to your approach to research?

Recommended reading

Freshwater, D. and Lees, J. (2008) *Practitioner-Based Research: Power, Discourse and Transformation*. London: Karnac.

This book approaches practitioner research from a broad healthcare perspective.

THREE   A cross-disciplinary and multi-method approach of multilingualism in psychotherapy

Jean-Marc Dewaele (Birkbeck College, University of London) & Beverley Costa (Mothertongue)

Jean-Marc Dewaele and Beverley Costa share their experience of doing mixed-methods research in a neglected area of psychotherapy.

- Multilingual therapy
- Mixed-method inquiry
- Quantitative and qualitative approaches
- Critical realism
- Positivism
- Social sciences
- Hypothesis
- Data collection
- Likert scale
- Factor analysis

Introductory comments: In this chapter Jean-Marc and Beverley will share their experiences of working with mixed methods in an under-researched area. As we shall see, Beverley's interest in larger sampling groups introduced her to some of the advantages of quantitative research. Together with Jean-Marc, who expands on the methods in detail in this chapter, Beverley was able to research multilingual therapy from several angles.

Practitioner perspective, by Beverley

In 2011, Mothertongue, a multi-ethnic counselling service (www.mother tongue.org.uk), decided to conduct research into the experiences of multilingual and monolingual therapists and counsellors working with multilingual clients. In order to provide a context for the research project carried out with Professor Jean-Marc Dewaele in 2012 (Costa and Dewaele 2012), I will attempt to share some of my dilemmas as a therapist and thinking about the way in which we conducted the research.

Mothertongue works therapeutically with clients from an average of 43 ethnic backgrounds and we deliver therapy in 15 languages. All of our therapists are multilingual and work regularly in all their languages with the clients. We are aware from our own practice that most models of therapy and most counselling and psychotherapy trainings do not attend to people's experiences of being multilingual. We also know from previous studies (Costa 2010; Nguyen 2012) that multilingual therapists can feel unsupported, unacknowledged and unprepared for working across languages, often in their mother tongue – a language in which they did not receive their training or their own counselling or therapy.

In order to strengthen the case for attention to be paid to this aspect of human experience, we decided that we needed to conduct research and gather robust evidence to support our claims that this is an area which merits further exploration.

So far in Mothertongue, we had argued for a form of research which is highly active and yields rapid results. Because of the pressing needs of the client group with whom we work, a long process of research-led practice can seem irrelevant, especially to those in need. We have therefore preferred to focus on action research methods which draw from educational provision, for example Kolb's Learning Cycle (1984) and Paolo Freire's (1990) emancipatory educational ideas.

As a therapist, it is not surprising that I am drawn to qualitative forms of research. My natural inclination is to avoid models which incline towards the generation of generalisations. In Jean-Marc's words, 'positivists believe that inquiries should be value free'. In psychotherapy, we focus on attending to individuals' voices and their subjective experiences. We are also aware of the impossibility of taking a neutral stance. Our very presence in the encounter shapes it in some way. This would incline me more towards qualitative methods, such as grounded theory, which value the meaning which can be generated from in-depth interviews with a small number of participants, while taking into account the social constructionist view that meaning is made through interaction with each other and with the social world. We encourage our clients and ourselves to take into account multiple perspectives as opposed to single versions of reality.

However, with qualitative research, sample sizes are often very small. We wanted to create as big a body of evidence as possible for this under-researched area to be taken seriously. I had no experience of quantitative forms of research and I had my own prejudices. This was an initial hurdle.

Developing an appreciation for number

Nevertheless I have developed an appreciation for the credibility which greater numbers of respondents, achievable through quantitative methods, can bring to one's research findings, especially in an under-researched area such as the experiences of multilinguals in therapy. It provides a starting point from which people can begin to debate ideas, challenge and create new models. A mixed-methods form of inquiry, which combines both quantitative and qualitative approaches, seems to fit well with reconciling and holding different perspectives. Holding tensions, after all, is what we therapists are constantly aiming to achieve in our work.

Reflection

Consider an area in your practice which could be explored both with a quantitative and qualitative approach.

In an attempt to find a way forward I started to look at the research being conducted in the field of Applied Linguistics into the emotional experiences of multilinguals. It struck me that the disciplines of Applied Linguistics and Psychotherapy could explore similar issues from different perspectives. Currently, they appear to be conducting these explorations in isolation from each other. For example, linguists may not focus on the relationship people have with their different languages and may focus more on the benefits of, say, the bilingual upbringing of children without reference to the parents' relationship with their languages.

Therapists tend to ignore the issue of whether multilinguals encode emotions differently and experience the world differently in different languages (Dewaele 2010). They may ignore the power issues played out in families: the potential for inclusion and exclusion via languages, which some family members share with each other (Karamati 2004).

It seemed important to try to bring those two disciplines together. I was very fortunate that Professor Jean-Marc Dewaele from the Applied Linguistics Department, at Birkbeck College, University of London also thought it was a good idea. With this collaboration, we were able to think about the research subject across disciplines. I was also able to learn a great deal about conducting quantitative research from a highly experienced practitioner. Without this collaboration I would never have dared to embark on a mixed-methods inquiry.

Critical Realism

This collaboration has fitted well with a Critical Realism approach (Bhaskar 1979). Through this approach, we have tried to refine our knowledge by using information and by observing and describing more fully that information via questionnaires and reflective conversations, in order to obtain as full and rich a description as possible. From that description, we have attempted an evaluative critique of what we have observed. We hope this will invite others to take part in that evaluative critique.

Ethical clearance

I want to end with a note about ethical clearance. At a recent conference a fellow delegate asked me why I thought there was a small but increasing body of research about multilingual therapists' experiences, but practically nothing available on the experiences of clients. My explanation for this is that the processes for gaining ethical clearance for medical research with patients and clients are so arduous that it is off-putting for researchers who, like ourselves, have very limited resources. We have had to consider how we approach this hurdle with our latest, subsequent research, which is focusing on patients' experiences. Our solution has been two-fold:

1. To use a non-intrusive method of data collection. We have therefore designed a questionnaire with open questions for people to share their stories if they wish to. So far, we have collected some very rich information from over 200 participants.
2. To recruit participants from our multilingual colleagues rather than from sources of identified patients. We have therefore sent the call for participants to all our multilingual colleagues without knowing which, if any, of them has received therapy. People can decide for themselves if they wish to answer the questionnaire, via Survey monkey, which is entirely anonymous.

If we had not made an effort to find a way of working with quantitative methods, then, with the limited resources we have, there would be no data from multilingual clients and their voices and their experiences would not be heard or taken into account in the research literature.

The researcher's perspective, by Jean-Marc

The cornerstones in quantitative research

Hatch and Farhady (1982: 1) defined the term 'research' as a systematic approach to answering questions. Farhady (2013: 1) highlights three key terms in this classic definition: 'a question, a systematic approach, and an answer', and observes that the debates in social sciences are not so much on the 'definition of the term "research" but on different interpretations of the key terms'.

The quantitative research method is based in the positivistic paradigm. Paradigms are based on four cornerstones: ontology, epistemology, methodology and axiology. Farhady (2013: 1) reminds us that:

> [Ontologically, positivists argue that] there is a real world, the reality of which is expressed in terms of the relationships among variables, and the extent of these relationships can be measured in a reliable and valid manner using a priori operational definitions.

Epistemologically, positivists place 'a premium on objective observation of the "real world" out there', continues Farhady (2013: 1). *Methodologically*, positivists prefer the use of deductive reasoning, 'a system for organizing known facts in order to reach a conclusion' (Farhady 2013: 2). The *conclusion* can only be true if the premise upon which it is based is true. As referred to in the previous chapter, positivists emphasise the importance of a priori hypotheses and theories. By manipulating at least one independent variable (i.e. 'the main or the cause variable which is under the control of the researcher' (Farhady 2013: 3)), the researcher measures its effect on a dependent variable, 'i.e. the variable that depends on, or changes as the result of, the manipulation of the independent variable', controlling for other moderator variables 'that may influence the outcome of the dependent variable without being necessarily manipulated' (Farhady 2013: 3). This procedure allows the researcher to establish valid cause–effect relationships and generalise them as laws.

The final cornerstone is *axiology*, which 'deals with the ethics and asks how moral a person a researcher should be in the world" (Farhady 2013: 2). Positivists believe that inquiries should be value free. Farhady 2013: 2) continues: 'In other words, the researcher's values, interpretations, feelings, and musings have no place in the positivist's view of scientific inquiry.'

Research questions, research design, data collection and analysis

The quantitative researcher starts, as Farhady (2013: 2) puts it, with a question 'which is formulated about the relationship between at least two variables'. A variable is 'any attribute that changes from person to person ..., place to place ..., or time to time'.

In social sciences, however, we mostly deal with abstract variables, 'that is, not directly observable or measureable but inferred from observations and measurements' (Farhady 2013: 2), with discrete or categorical variables, such as gender, and continuous variables can take any value, such as frequencies, number of languages known. At the heart of the investigation lies the research questions 'about the relationship between the variables to indicate either a cause–effect relationship or just ... togetherness between them'.

Once the research question is formulated with well-defined variables (allowing replication), 'it is converted into a research hypothesis to be tested. A hypothesis is a tentative statement about the outcome of research and can take two forms: null and alternative' (Farhady 2013: 3).

A null hypothesis H0, continues Farhady (2013: 3), 'is generally stated in the form that the manipulation of the independent variable will not have an effect upon the dependent variable'. The alternative hypothesis 'stipulates an effect, either positive or negative, of the independent variable on the dependent variable'.

Once the research hypothesis is formulated, the researcher chooses a systematic approach, a research design, to test the research hypothesis. The quality of the design will depend on many factors, including the nature of the research question, the type and number of variables, the number and groups of subjects participating in research, and the type of collected data. Combining these to form an efficient design will optimise the outcome of the research.

The data collection is the next stage. This is of crucial importance 'because the validity of the findings of research will depend very much on the quality of the collected data' (Farhady 2013: 8). Farhady continues: 'Therefore, great care should be exercised in selecting appropriate instruments for data collection.'

Statistics will be needed to analyse the data (Dancey and Reidy 2011). The quantitative researcher will have to interpret the findings and discuss their implications for improving the theory and their applications to practice. It is, for instance, important to underline that 'the validity of the findings depends on the validity of research' (Farhady 2013: 8). In other words, statistical significance does not automatically lead to a firm law. It is better to be careful in making conclusions, avoiding strong and sweeping statements because of the inherent limitations of any research design.

The strengths and weaknesses of quantitative research

The quantitative approach has major strengths: it is 'systematic, rigorous, focused, and tightly controlled, involving precise measurement and producing reliable and replicable data that is generalisable to other contexts' (Dörnyei 2007: 34). However, quantitative methods have two main weaknesses. Dörnyei (2007: 35) concludes that:

- First, 'they average out responses across the whole observed group of participants, and by working with concepts of averages it is impossible to do justice to the subjective variety of an individual life'.
- Second, they 'have a rather limited general exploratory capacity because they cannot easily uncover reasons for particular patterns or the dynamics underlying a situation or phenomenon'.

> **Reflection**
>
> Consider the strengths and weaknesses of quantitative research with reference to your potential research interest.

Mixed-methods research

The obvious way to overcome the limitations of quantitative research is by including a qualitative component to the research design: 'I have also experienced again and again how much richer data we can obtain in a well-conducted and analysed qualitative study than even in a large-scale questionnaire survey' (Dörnyei 2007: 47).

The integration of qualitative and quantitative analyses is called mixed-methods research and is still in its infancy (Tashakkori and Teddlie, 2010). Leech and Dellinger (2013: 6) underline that 'it is important to consider validity evidence when conducting mixed methods research so that studies are rigorous and results and inferences are defensible'.

Rather than talking about the 'validity' of mixed-methods research, Teddlie and Tashakkori (2009) propose 'inference quality', defined as a combination of design quality (i.e. whether the study adheres to best practice) and interpretive rigor (i.e. how well the results can be trusted).

Dewaele (2010) has argued that for research into multilinguals' feelings, language choices and perceptions, it is important to combine quantitative and qualitative data. The former were obtained through the use of an online questionnaire comprising closed questions (with 5-point Likert scales) and open questions, which allowed participants to add their own unique observations. More than 1,500 participants responded via social media and email and filled out the questionnaire. As they came from all over the world, ranging in age from teenagers to elderly participants, the ecological validity of the resulting database was solid. The fact that the sample was not a representative sample of the general population (having a high proportion of female, highly educated multilinguals) was not a problem, because this self-selected sample of highly linguistically and pragmatically aware multilinguals was best able to produce high-quality information. Wilson and Dewaele (2010) reported that self-selected participants are more likely to make an effort to provide complete, accurate and honest feedback.

One crucial element is obviously to use a good research instrument, where the closed questions have clear items with Likert scales, and where the open questions are unambiguous (Dörnyei 2010).

The statistical analysis allowed the identification of general patterns in the data, namely the effect of sociobiographical variables, language learning history, current linguistic practice and psychological variables on the dependent variables (Dewaele 2010). Once these patterns had been established, the quantitative data were complemented with inter-view data from 20 multilinguals who had filled out the questionnaire. This allowed more in-depth probing of reported linguistic behaviour and attitudes, and a better understanding of the unique combination of individual, social, pragmatic and cultural reasons linked to the dependent variables.

Costa and Dewaele (2012)

Costa and Dewaele (2012) followed a similar approach: an online questionnaire was designed, which was aimed specifically at psychotherapists. It included closed questions (with Likert scales) related to the participants' beliefs, attitudes and practices.

A previous version of the questionnaire had been submitted to four experts (two psychologists and two applied linguists), who rated each of the original 89 items on a 5-point Likert scale (ranging from 'poor validity' to 'strong validity') and commented on them. Then the questionnaire was pilot-tested with 10 therapists. The final version was cut to 27 items and put online on Survey Monkey (see Figure 3.1).

As a rule of thumb, filling out questionnaires should not exceed 10 to 15 minutes (Dörnyei 2010). The items were statements, and the participants were asked to express their degree of disagreement or agreement with the statement. For example: *I think that therapists with bilingual skills are able to understand clients in a different way than therapists who are monolingual.* And: *It is easier to express strong feelings and emotions in a second language.* And: *From*

Tell us to what extent you agree with the following statements regardless of whether you have had therapy with a multilingual therapist. If you have not had therapy with a multilingual therapist, we are still interested in your ideas.

	Strongly disagree	Disagree	Neutral	Agree	Strongly agree
1. I avoid certain topics when talking to a therapist with whom I do not share a first language (L1).	O	O	O	O	O
2. I avoid certain topics when talking to a therapist with whom I share a L1.	O	O	O	O	O
3. Therapists with whom I share a first language relate differently from therapists with whom I do not share a L1.	O	O	O	O	O

Figure 3.1   Example of Likert scale questioning, taken from Costa and Dewaele (2012)

my experience, I feel that levels of empathy between clients and therapists are affected by the language in which the therapy takes place. The instruction was: *Tell us to what extent you agree with the following statements (Strongly disagree, Disagree, Neutral, Agree, Strongly Agree).*

Activity

Consider how you might phrase some of your research questions using a Likert scale format. Would your research lend itself to this kind of questioning?

Participants were recruited through Beverley's contacts in the profession. The questionnaire was anonymous but participants could leave an email address if they agreed to be interviewed on the issues covered in the questionnaire.

The main independent variable was the therapist's language knowledge (mono- or multilingual). As this was one among many sociobiographical background questions (other questions included gender, age, nationality, language history, present language use, and theoretical orientation in their therapeutic work), the participants could not guess that mono-/multilingualism was the main independent variable.

Factor analysis

An exploratory factor analysis, using a principal components analysis (PCA) was performed on the 27 items, followed by an independent t-test comparing the factor scores of the monolingual and multilingual therapists. The most difficult part in the PCA is the interpretation of the solution. In this case, it was a four-factor solution accounting for 41% of the variance. By comparing the five items with strong positive and one item with a strong negative loading on the first dimension, it was determined that the first factor (with an eigenvalue of 4.7 and explaining 17% of variance) reflected therapists' attunement towards their bilingual clients (Attunement versus Collusion).

Individual factor scores on the various dimensions were used as the dependent variables. An independent t-test showed that the 18 monolingual therapists differed significantly from their 83 bilingual or multilingual peers on the first dimension (Attunement versus Collusion). The multilingual therapists are situated more towards the Attunement end of the dimension compared to the monolingual therapists.

The second factor was named 'Shared understanding versus Acting on assumptions' (explaining 9% of variance). The third and fourth factors reflected 'Freedom of expression versus Difficulty of challenging', and 'The distancing effect of the second language versus The advantage of a shared language', explaining an additional 15% of variance. Individual factor scores on the various dimensions were used as the dependent variables.

Our null hypothesis and the outcome of our study

The null hypothesis was that monolingual therapists would not differ from their multilingual peers. An independent t-test showed that the 18 monolingual therapists differed significantly from their 83 multilingual peers on the first dimension, and hence that the null hypothesis could be rejected. The multilingual therapists were situated closer to the Attunement end of the dimension compared to the monolingual therapists, who were closer to the Collusion end of the dimension. No statistically significant differences between both groups emerged on the three other dimensions, meaning the null hypothesis stood firm. Armed with that knowledge, Beverley interviewed one monolingual and two multilingual therapists and managed to probe their views and uncover possible causes for the patterns that had emerged in the quantitative analysis.

Recommended reading

Dörnyei, Z. (2007) *Research Methods in Applied Linguistics: Quantitative, Qualitative and Mixed Methodologies.* Oxford: Oxford University Press.

This book gives a comprehensive overview of the various stages of qualitative and quantitative investigations from collecting the data to presenting the results.

FOUR   What is evidence-based research?

Randomised controlled trials, systemic reviews and meta-analysis are some of the frequently used terms in today's research about therapy. This chapter looks closely at evidence-based research, focusing on objectivity.

- Evidence
- NICE guidance
- Systematic review
- Meta-analysis
- Cochrane library
- Randomised controlled trials (RCTs)
- CORE-OM
- Mixed methods
- Positivist realism

In the previous chapter, Beverley Costa and Jean-Marc Dewaele explored the benefits with mixed-methods research. Jean-Marc also explained the principles behind quantitative research, for instance with regard to their null hypothesis, factor analysis, etc. In this chapter, we will expand on quantitative research with reference to evidence-based research.

'Empirically supported', 'evidence-based' methods and 'treatments' are, as suggested, guiding concepts in official guidelines about therapy. There is in this sense, as suggested earlier, a shift in the terminology surrounding psychotherapy. Terms like 'diagnosis', 'disorder' and 'solution focused' may have been reserved for more medically informed frameworks, but are now part of an overriding discourse about issues linked to therapeutic processes. The so-called NICE guidance are standards set by the National Institute for Health and Care Excellence, providing healthcare guidelines for the 'NHS, Local Authorities, employers, voluntary groups and anyone else involved in delivering care or promoting wellbeing' (www.nice.org.uk/guidance, 2012). The NICE guidance is a driving force behind evidence-based research. NICE guidelines for psychological treatments are being legitimised on the basis of the aim to increase access to psychological treatments guided by evidence-based research. The evidence-based research is guided by a hierarchy of 'trustworthiness', where the randomised control trial is the 'golden standard'.

Questions in evidence-based research can typically be answered with a 'yes' or 'no'. *Does therapy help? Does orientation matter?* These kinds of questions often involve a focus on 'efficacy', which means 'the potential to bring about a desired effect' (Cooper 2008: 17):

> To show that psychological therapies are 'efficacious' – that is, that they bring about a desired effect – it is necessary to compare changes in clients who have undergone therapy; what is a called a control group. This could be people who are waiting for therapy or people who are receiving treatment. If, in this comparison, the people who have therapy change more than a similar group of people who do not have therapy ... then we can be fairly certain that the therapy, and no other factor, is responsible for the changes.

Activity

To what extent do the NICE guidelines impact on your practice?

If you are not already familiar with the guidelines, we encourage you to look at some of the information that is available for download. You can download documents from www.nice.org.uk/guidance for recommendations on the identification, treatment and management of mental health issues within the NHS and Local Authorities. For instance, identification and pathways to care regarding common mental health disorders can be found at: www.nice.org.uk/guidance/CG123.

The hierarchy on which evidence-based practice is based refers to 'systematic reviews and randomised controlled trials at the top and qualitative studies at the bottom', as listed by Aveyard and Sharp (2009: 73) below:

- Systematic reviews and meta-analyses
- Randomised controlled trial
- Cohort studies, case-controlled studies
- Surveys
- Case reports
- Qualitative studies
- Expert opinion and anecdotal opinion

This puts experiments and the deductive forms of reasoning to the forefront. As referred to earlier, deductive reasoning starts with some form of prediction or a 'hypothesis or a measurable statement', which takes the research, as Moule and Hek (2011: 63) explain, 'from the specific to the general':

In research terms [moving from the specific to the general] means a prediction is made of the presence, or not, of a difference or a relationship between two or more factors (usually referred to as variables). The prediction is made through a hypothesis or measurable statement that can be deduced from a theory. The prediction will then be tested. The results of the research will either support the prediction or not, thereby confirming the theory or not.

To recap, in this sense deductive approaches rely on:

- a theory to 'give the study a focus', and

- needs a previously tested data-collecting tool to gather information, from a

- representative sample of a research population

- the results usually require 'rigorous statistical testing in which the possibility of these results occurring by chance will be demonstrated and discussed'. (Moule and Hek 2011: 148)

Randomised control trial model

The randomised control trial (RCT) model is regarded as the most 'trustworthy' form of evidence. RCT is designed to provide an approach that is as neutral and objective as possible. Sackett et al. (2000: 1) conclude:

Evidence based medicine is the conscientious, explicit, and judicious use of current best evidence in making decisions about the care of individual patients. ... By best available external clinical evidence we mean clinically relevant research, often from the basic sciences of medicine, but especially from patient centred clinical research into the accuracy and precision of diagnostic tests (including the clinical examination), the power of prognostic markers, and the efficacy and safety of therapeutic, rehabilitative, and preventive regimens.

Transparency and accountability can have a refreshing input on stuffy consultation rooms, and conveys hopes that mind-related issues can be cured in the same way that broken legs, mumps and measles can be cured. Assessment forms, evaluations sheets and written contracts are some of the means of capturing the therapeutic process.

Activity

Describe your role as a therapist.

- What do you actually do?
- Describe a key characteristic of your therapy work.
- How important are assessment forms and evaluation sheets in your practice? What other means of negotiating and monitoring the goals in your practice do you use?
- How do you measure progress?

The RCT model involves the comparison of a randomly chosen 'case group', which is exposed to a certain intervention, with a 'control group', which is subjected to a benign or placebo intervention. In the following case study, Aveyard and Sharp (2009) illustrate the process of conducting an RCT in a weight loss programme.

Case study

Participants are allocated into the different treatments groups of the trial at random. ... Once each treatment group in the trial has been randomly allocated, the groups are considered as equal, and the intervention treatment is given to group one. The second group receives either the standard treatment or no treatment or placebo. ... The groups are then observed and the difference between the groups in terms of weight loss is monitored. ... (Aveyard and Sharp 2009: 60)

As is typical in so-called deductive reasoning, there is a hypothesis guiding the experiment and falsification of the hypothesis is the means of validating the outcome. Aveyard and Sharp (2009: 60) continue:

[A] null hypothesis is usually stated when an RCT is designed. The null hypothesis states that there is no difference between the two groups. The aim of the RCT is to determine whether the null hypothesis can be confirmed or rejected. If the results show that there is a difference between the control group and the intervention group, the null hypothesis can be rejected.

Some of the steps for conducting an RCT for a weight loss programme may be as follows (Aveyard and Sharp 2009: 60):

- A poster will be sited in a weight loss clinic, inviting people who are interested in entering a trial to compare weight loss treatments.
- Interested people will respond to the advertisement, and those who fit the inclusion criteria will become the sample population. They will randomly be allocated into two groups.
- Group one receives the new weight loss intervention strategy.
- Group two receive standard clinic treatment.
- The rate of weight loss is compared between the two groups.
- Any differences will be attributed to the different treatments which the groups received.

Is there a general 'cure' for depression? Can symptoms, such as hopelessness or showing little interest in pleasure, be approached in terms of 'real' entities, such as the symptoms of mumps, measles or pregnancy? It certainly becomes more complex when we deal with feelings and states of mind. When do, say, feelings of hopelessness and a lack of pleasure reflect 'depression'? Consider, for instance, the references to depression, cited from the NICE guidance below:

Be alert to possible depression (particularly in people with a past history of depression, possible somatic symptoms of depression or a chronic physical health problem with associated functional impairment) and consider asking people who may have depression two questions, specifically:

During the last month, have you often been bothered by feeling down, depressed or hopeless?

During the last month, have you often been bothered by having little interest or pleasure in doing things?

If a person answers 'yes' to either of the above questions consider depression and follow the recommendations for assessment (see section 1.3.2). (NICE 2007)

Reflection

Different modalities tend to approach 'depression' differently. Psychoanalytically inspired therapy often regards depression as suppressed anger. How does your modality inform you to define and approach a problem like 'depression'?

When we explore research inspired by the RCT model, we will find bite-size 'certainties' about, for instance, depression and postnatal problems, depression and age or, as in the example below, depression and exercise. The next case study illustrates the role of meta-analysis, systematic review and randomised control trials.

Case study

Meta-analysis and systematic review

The term 'meta-analysis' refers to the process of comparing multiple studies that have investigated common problems. In evidence-based practice (EBP), meta-analysis comprises the highest form of evidence. Practitioners can access these through a free online library called the Cochrane Library (www.thecochranelibrary.com/view/0/index.html).

We have already explored the issue of the literature review in the context of practice-based research. The evidence-based approach to literature reviews differs slightly to the practice-based approach. Strictly speaking, only literature reviews which involve studies which have been 'pre-appraised for scientific validity' qualify as reviews 'based on best evidence'. Aveyard and Sharp (2009: 56) conclude that although the terms 'systematic review' usually refer to the 'Cochrane Collaboration method' of reviewing, it is sometimes referred to in literature reviews that adopt less rigorous methods. The kind of literature review that we will look at in Chapter 6 by Simon du Plock tends to come closer to what in evidence-based research is referred to as 'narrative reviews'. These will, according to Aveyard and Sharp (2009: 56), have less focused research questions, a less focused searching strategy and will neither be guided by 'clear methods of appraisal or synthesis of literature'. They are 'not easily repeatable' either.

Sacket et al. (2000: 32, 30, 48) recommend all practitioners to 'invest in evidence-based databases', and they go so far as to suggest that we 'burn' traditional textbooks if they are over one year old because they will no longer be up to date and will fail to comply with the scientific validity criteria:

> Burn your (traditional) textbooks. We begin with textbooks only to dismiss them. If the pages of textbooks smelled like decomposing garbage when they got out of date, the unsmelly bits could be useful. Unfortunately, there's no way to tell what is up to date and what is not in most texts. ... Having made the bold claim if we were to burn the textbooks we would begin to see a phoenix of sorts arising from the ashes. For a textbook to be dependable in the modern era

- It should be revised ... at least once a year
- It should be heavily referenced ...
- The evidence in support of statement should be selected according to explicit principles of evidence. (Sacket et al. 2000: 48)

Reflection

How many of your textbooks would you have to 'burn' to comply with the criteria of using work-related literature which is revised and updated yearly? Look in some of your favourite books and check the year of publication at the front of the book on the copyright page.

Sacket et al. (2000: 32) refer to electronic databases such as the Cochrane Library, MEDLINE, PsycINFO, etc. Typically these databases contain research which is 'clinically pre-screened' and 'pre-appraised for scientific validity'. Sacket et al. (2000: 32, 34, 48) continue:

> Although not integrated around clinical problem areas in the consistent way of textbooks, current best evidence from specific studies of clinical problems can be found in an increasing number of electronic databases. ... The best of these at present is Evidence-based Medicine Review (EBMR) [which combines] several electronic databases, including the Cochrane Database of Systematic Reviews, Bets Evidence, Evidence-Based Mental Health, etc. ... [which] contain only studies that have been pre-appraised for scientific validity and pre-screened for clinical relevance. Thus, you can select to skip the report's methodology.

Activity

Go to the Cochrane Library on the link below, tap in your research topic and look at some of the research which comes up: www.thecochranelibrary.com/view/0/index.html.

- How do these studies relate to your research interest?
- Is there any pattern or common theme among the studies?
- Do you think there is sufficient variation for reflexivity and for 'pitting' contrasting understandings against each other?
- Consider the pros and cons of the systemic and the traditional 'narrative' literature review.

Evidence-based practice and practice-based evidence

Evidence-based research lends itself to deductive reasoning. The 'null hypothesis', mentioned earlier in context of the weight loss programme, is an example of deductive reasoning. It predicts that there will be no relationship between the variables which are measured. In the case of the weight loss research, the null hypothesis suggested that there would be no difference between the two sample groups.

Although practice-based evidence does not exclude evidence-based studies, Barkham et al. (2010: 37) conclude that 'while RCTs [randomised controlled trials] can be construed as applying multiple layers of filters to ensure a very precise target data set, practice-based studies relax these filters with the specific purpose of trying to reflect the activity of routine practice'. Practice-based studies are 'molded to reflect everyday clinical practice' with an 'aim to capture data drawn from routine practice', as Barkham et al. (2010: 39) put it.

Practice-based research is common in studies linked to arts and design, where integrating creative processes and artistic strategies into the academic classification system has been an issue. The implications of research that takes place in real life and is carried out by practitioners have given rise to new concepts and methods, which offer exciting options for understanding more about the richness and complexity of life. We will return to the issue about practice-based research being characterised by its 'situatedness' (Costley et al. 2010: 1). Situated knowledge is knowledge specific to a particular situation. On an immediate, practical level, it becomes obvious, perhaps, that the unique personal, professional and organisational involvement of an 'insider' researcher will impact the way a piece of research is undertaken.

The origins of the term 'situated knowledge' is often linked to the feminist, Donna Haraway (1991), who asserts that knowledge is always embedded in language, culture or tradition. As we shall see as we begin to unpick the concept of reflexivity later on in this book, Haraway's (1991: 194) guiding questions fit in well in practice-based research with a reflexive approach:

Histories of science may be powerfully told as histories of the technologies. These technologies are ways of life, social orders, practices of visualization. Technologies are skilled practices. How to see? Where to see from? What limits the visions? What to see for? Whom to see with? Who gets to have more than one point of view? Who gets blinkered? Who wears blinkers? Who interprets the visual field?

Practice-based research encourages practitioners from all walks of life to engage in an ongoing evaluation of both their own and others' practice. It suggests that we generate knowledge with an openness for nuances and by using a greater variety of methods than the evidence-based approaches allow for, while adhering to the typical emphasis on transparency and accountability that evidence-based practice calls for. As already mentioned, practice-based evidence 'starts with the practitioner'. This does not exclude evidence-based research. The overriding aim in practice-based research is for the practitioner 'to effect change with their client ... regardless of [the practitioner's] orientation ... organisation or context within which they work' (Barkham et al. 2010: 335). Barkham et al. (2010: 214) refer to the CORE-system (Clinical Outcomes in Routine Evaluation) as an example of where practice-based and evidence-based research marries well:

[W]hen used optimally, the [CORE] system reflects patient centred practice as its best. Not only do clients provide responses to the measure items, but practitioners and patients work collaboratively to understand and interpret the patient's progress chart ... and recognize in real time when progress is being made or, if not, review alternative strategies.

Barkham et al. (2005: 2) explain the content of the patient self-report measure CORE-OM form below:

The CORE-OM comprises 34 items addressing domains of subjective well-being (4 items), symptoms (12 items), functioning (12 items) and risk (6 items; 4 'risk to self' items and 2 'risk to others' items). Within the symptom domain 'item clusters' address anxiety (4 items), depression (4 items), physical problems (2 items) and trauma (2 items). The functioning domain item clusters address general functioning (4 items), close relationships (4 items) and social relationships (4 items). Items are scored on a five-point scale from 0 ('not at all') to 4 ('all the time'). Half of the items focus on low-intensity problems (e.g. 'I feel anxious/nervous') and half focus on high-intensity problems (e.g. 'I feel panic/terror'). Eight items are keyed positively.

Reflection

Many practitioners choose to assess their clients with a measuring tool like the CORE-OM. In the case study below, the earlier mentioned Alan Priest refers to some of the benefits in his practice. To what extent would using measuring systems fit in with your modality and clinical practice?

Case study

Alan Priest (2013: 192) writes:

[Eleven] clients were recruited to the study and completed a CORE-OM assessment at the start of therapy. They completed a further CORE-OM assessment at the end of therapy, just prior to their post therapy qualitative interview. This is common practice in evaluation (Stiles 2010: 649). Data from these assessments were entered into a Microsoft Excel workbook which I created to provide a simple representation of pre- and post-therapy scores in graphical format, as well as the basis for simple analysis of change across all four measures obtained by the instrument. Again, I emphasise that this is part of my normal way of working with clients.

The development of the Clinical Outcomes in Routine Evaluation Outcome Measure (CORE-OM) started in 1993, following a conference for the Mental Health Foundation, after which a multi-centre collaborative group, led by Michael Barkham, won a competitive tender to develop an outcome measure for use within the NHS.

CORE-OM is used widely in both primary and secondary care settings as a way of routinely monitoring client outcomes from different types of

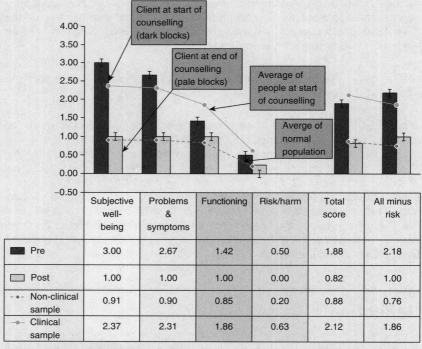

	Subjective well-being	Problems & symptoms	Functioning	Risk/harm	Total score	All minus risk
Pre	3.00	2.67	1.42	0.50	1.88	2.18
Post	1.00	1.00	1.00	0.00	0.82	1.00
Non-clinical sample	0.91	0.90	0.85	0.20	0.88	0.76
Clinical sample	2.37	2.31	1.86	0.63	2.12	1.86

Figure 4.1 Comparison of pre- and post-scores for FS with non-clinical ('normal') and clinical ('pathology') samples of 1084 and 863 respectively

counselling and psychotherapy. CORE-OM materials are freely available to download – an advantage for self-funding researchers such as myself. Analysis based on large samples has demonstrated reliability and convergent validity against longer and less general measures and good sensitivity to change. ... The results of over 100 research projects demonstrating the efficacy of CORE-OM have been published in peer-reviewed academic publications .... CORE-OM has been shown to be highly correlated with the Beck Depression Inventory in routine clinical practice.

The term 'real-life research' involves at some stage some serious thinking about what we consider to be real. Do we, for instance, hope to contribute with something definite about reality, such as the actual number of cars that pass through red lights in the traffic light scenario earlier mentioned? Or do we hope to contribute with knowledge about people's perception or experience of, for instance, traffic lights. A qualitative study may highlight how drivers' relationship to authority is being transferred into their traffic light behaviour. Perhaps some drivers connect the red light with a dominant parent or teacher from the past and feel the need to rebel. Other drivers may hear a tender, caring voice from the past explaining why they should be cautious and look after oneself and others as they approach the lights. Both types of information are valid and important. As we will explore further, later in this book, our underpinning philosophy about reality will invariably be reflected through our choice of research methods.

The RCT model has, as suggested earlier, developed from the natural scientific experiment model with its focus on cause and effect. This requires tangible factors which can be measured. A common example is the testing of the effectiveness of a new vaccine. The cause and effect scenario becomes more complex when dealing with psychological treatment. For instance, is it ethical to expose clients to interventions which they don't know about as, strictly speaking, randomised control trials suggest? Also, symptoms such as hopelessness, lack of pleasure and anxiety are difficult to measure. Are we talking about a symptom which exists independently of our perception – i.e. something which can be studied within a realist framework – or are we working with people's perception of reality, within an idealist or relativist epistemology? The space between so-called naive 'realism' and 'idealism' creates a framework which invites us to consider the implications of our assumptions.

Marks (2002: 9–10) positions the evidence-based approaches within the epistemological stance, called 'positivist realism'. Positive realism assumes an epistemological stance which 'views science as a mirror of nature that reveals the truth' and where 'the researcher's task is to make accurate observations about objective reality'. Marks (2002: 9–10) expands on this theme below:

EBP is an adaptation of epistemology and methodology derived from the natural sciences and applied to fields of clinical medicine, healthcare and education.

The currently accepted epistemological assumptions of EBP are a form of positivist realism or 'positive realism' (PR). Positive realism has been traced back to the philosophy of Descartes, who proposed that we have direct knowledge of subjective, mental reality ('I think, therefore I am'), but must derive our knowledge of objective, physical reality through observation. ... The researcher's task is to make accurate observations about objective reality, ensuring that error and bias are eliminated by isolating variables in order to be able to identify cause–effect relationships. Thus PR [positivist realist] views science as a mirror of nature that reveals the truth.

Practice-based research and the 'messiness' of life

Practice-based research emerges from experiences developed through active engagement with a wide range of 'real-life' settings. The basic claim for practice-based research is that the inquiry, as Robson (2002: 10) puts it, 'can be of help in gaining an understanding of the human situations and its manifestation in an office, factory, school, hospital or any other environment, and in initiating sensible change and development'. This means, continues Robson (2002: 10), that we invariably will do research under 'relatively poorly controlled and generally "messy" situations'. Significant for practice-based research is, as Costley et al. (2010: 1) argue, its 'situatedness': there is an 'interplay between the researcher as a person, the particular set of circumstances which the researcher is positioned in and the overall context; the where, when and general background'. The 'organizational, professional and personal context will affect the way a piece of research and development is undertaken', conclude Costley et al. (2010: 1). The practice-based research aims to include rather than exclude the complexity of real life – be it on an organizational or a personal, unique level. Practice-based research is, as Barkham et al. (2010: 335) explain: 'pluralistic with regards to research methods'. It tends, however, to argue for the need to broaden the definition of evidence, where idiographic and inductive reasoning to problems are included, and pay attention to unique, individual experiences and provide space for unanticipated themes to emerge.

Recommended reading

Hoffman, T., Bennett, S. and Del Mar, C. (eds) (2009) *Evidence-Based Practice across the Health Professions*. Chatswood: Elsevier.

This book is recommended to readers with an interest in evidence-based research in context of different strands of healthcare.

FIVE Formulating the research question

This chapter focuses on identifying and articulating the research question. Using different real-life examples, we will encourage you to formulate a research question of your own.

- Research question
- Coherence
- Focus
- Framework
- Participants

Finding your niche

It has been argued in this book that the purpose with research is almost always complex and multilayered. To be authentic, congruent and honest can sometimes feel that we are complicating things even further. How *can* we describe the root of the question, especially if research is assumed to become part of the discovery?

To clearly identify and articulate the research question is often, as Moule and Hek (2011: 78) argue, 'one of the most difficult stages in the research process'. Finlay and Ballinger (2006) concur, saying how difficult it often is to identify and articulate the research question:

> The research question is the most important statement we have to make about our subject matter and the mode of investigation. It is also the most difficult. [It is easy] for the novice researcher to drift into method, deciding strategies for data collection without determining what they want to study, why and with what epistemological perspective. (Finlay and Ballinger 2006: 34)

It is ultimately a question of identifying a niche within a massive area. We are unlikely to embark on research in a well-known area; the point is usually to deal with something that is either overwhelming or incomprehensible, or at least yet relatively unknown. It is with some reluctance that we have to narrow, almost 'box in', this great mystery into one, or if we're lucky, two sentences. As a rule of thumb, it is always better to start narrow and branch out, rather than to promise too much and deliver too little.

Say a lot about a little problem

The first step is therefore, as Finlay and Ballinger (2006: 34) put it, 'to select a well-defined topic of manageable size ... the aim should be to say a lot about a *little* problem'. One solution is to focus on a question which we think our research can actually answer, which is where the 'saying a lot about a little problem' comes in. As an example, Melanie Hopkins' research concerns a huge problem area, namely what it is like to work in a forensic psychiatric hospital.

Case study

Melanie Hopkins (2012: 18) explains some background to her personal and professional experience to the research:

> I am employed within the Priory Secure Services, specifically Thornford Park Hospital. Thornford Park is a low and medium secure Forensic Psychiatric Hospital. The building and secure surrounding grounds offer superb internal and external therapeutic and recreational facilities. The accommodation comprises 123 beds, low and medium secure, offering high quality, individualised care, treatment and rehabilitation for men aged 18+ who are detained under the Mental Health Act (1983) and difficult to place in National Health Service (NHS) facilities. There are 65 low secure rehab beds in four wards, 23 medium secure beds in two wards, a 10 bed ward specialising in short-term, enhanced low secure assessment, and a 17 bed ward for patients who are elderly and physically frail. The hospital also incorporates rehabilitation flats with rooms for seven patients to live with greater independence prior to discharge. Staff at the hospital cares for patients with a wide range of mental health issues, including those with personality disorders. ... My role within Thornford Park involves chairing the monthly Recovery Steering Group meeting, which leads on the implementation of the Recovery philosophy and model throughout the Hospital. This role involves developing and presenting staff and patient Recovery training and initiatives. Further, I am employed as a Forensic Psychotherapist, within the Psychology Department. I provide consultation to staff on the assessment and psychotherapeutic intervention of 27 patients. Together with other members of the hospital, I provide therapeutic intervention in the form of individual and group-based psycho-education and psychotherapeutic intervention to the patients within the hospital. Within the role of ward-based psychologist, I also provide staff support in the form of individual and group-based staff working in a Forensic environment [who] are exposed to patients who have committed serious psychological harm, sexual/violence against another or themselves.

Melanie adopts a formal, almost understated tone in her personal reflection. The careful selection of words indicates, however, the pressure involved in her role as therapist and supervisor for staff who are 'exposed to patients who have committed serious psychological harm, sexual/violence against another or themselves'.

Finlay and Balinger (2006: 337) suggest that the research question should indicate the purpose of the study, a broad methodology and 'whether the study aims to influence policy, practice or theory'. Quoting Punch, Finlay and Balinger (2006: 36) refer to 'five roles for the research question'. It should:

- give coherence and direction to the research project
- identify its boundaries
- provide a focus for the investigation
- offer a framework for writing up the project
- indicate which data will be needed to answer it.

Another way of addressing the process towards formulating a manageable problem is in terms of 'the five Ws'. Dawson (2009: 6) lists the following Ws as 'a useful way of remembering the important questions to ask':

- **What?** Sum up, in one sentence only, your research, advises Dawson (2009: 6): 'If you are unable to do this, the chances are your research topic is too broad, ill thought out or too obscure'.
- **Why?** Why are you interested in the topic? Have you found a gap in the literature? Are you trying to obtain funding? Does your research involve finding out whether there is a demand for your service? Will your research facilitate decision making?
- **Who?** Who are your participants? What type of people do you need to contact?
- **Where?** This involves geographical issue and resources, for instance travel expenses and time. What about the venue? Are you doing interviews or focus groups?
- **When?** What kind of time scale have you got in mind?

Case study

The guiding question for Melanie's study became 'What is the staff experience of hope in a forensic psychiatric hospital?' Hopkins (2012: 12–16) explains her overall aims, methodological considerations and the potential impact of the study as follows:

The study aims to gain an in-depth understanding of the experience of hope for staff within a forensic psychiatric hospital utilising a qualitative

(Continued)

(Continued)

study focused upon the experiences of staff, in order to keep the sample homogeneous. [It involves] participants from Psychiatry, Psychology, Occupational Therapy and Nursing, with a view toward exploring and utilising those thoughts, feelings and behaviours which can be helpful in order to drive organisational change toward mutually increasing both staff and patients' experience of hope. The Hope Theory was utilised as the framework for eliciting an understanding of hope, including associated goals, pathways and barriers. ...

A qualitative, rather than quantitative, research approach has been chosen for this project, as 'hope' – as it appears in the literature – is individualistic and better appreciated via an approach that can capture experiential insights and emotional reactions. In using Phenomenology as the epistemological position, 'we are assuming that our data will permit us access to a reasonably rich and reflective level of personal account, telling us something of a person's orientation towards the world and how they make sense of this' (Smith et al., 2009: 46). ... Whilst quantitative research has enabled a great deal of progress, it also has limitations. For example, since such research often utilises structured reporting methods, participants can only comment upon what they are asked to respond to, and this may produce a fragmented picture. ... With this in mind, and considering how the particular research question of this study may best be addressed, it was decided to adopt a qualitative methodology. Such an approach has the advantage of allowing in-depth and detailed study of phenomena that are not easily quantifiable, as in this study of 'staff experience of hope'. A further advantage was that such an approach allows for the emergence of unanticipated findings (Barker, Pistrang & Elliot, 2002). ...

The findings from this research project will drive organisational change in the following ways: to provide an Electronic Learning Module on the Recovery Model for all Priory Secure Service Staff to complete on an annual compulsory basis, thereby increasing staff understanding of Recovery and role of hope within their own lives.

Approaching therapy from the clients' side

Another approach to psychiatric problems is taken by Roz D'Ombraine Hewitt, in her research into the 'lived experience' of integrative psychotherapy for individuals diagnosed with schizophrenia/schizo-affective disorder.

Case study

D'Ombraine Hewitt (2012: 12) writes about her research as follows:

> The aim of this study was to investigate the 'lived experience' of integra-
> tive psychotherapy for individuals who have been diagnosed as being on
> the S/S-AD spectrum and to answer the research question:
>
> How does the experience of H-I [Humanistic/integrative] counselling
> impact upon the recovery of individuals who have been diagnosed as be-
> ing on the S/S-AD spectrum?
>
> Research objectives:
>
> • To further my learning of recovery from S/S-AD and use this to gain fresh
>   knowledge and thereby improve my work as a practitioner-researcher
> • To contribute to the literature and practice of counselling/psychotherapy on
>   recovery from S/S-AD
> • To further disseminate my research findings through my 'products', e.g.
>   workshops, presentation and performances of my drama-documentary.

Again, the background to the study is multilayered. Roz approaches therapy with an emphasis on 'meaning-making' processes and personal motivations. She suggests that we distinguish therapeutic outcomes in terms of
medical and personal recovery:

> The concept of *personal recovery* emerged from the expertise of individuals
> with lived experience of mental illness. *In contrast to medical recovery*, which
> involves a person being free of symptoms and 'getting back to normal', per-
> sonal recovery is: 'The unique, self-determined process of reclaiming meaning
> and purpose through living a hopeful, satisfying and contributing life, even with
> the limitations caused by illness or disability' (D'Ombraine Hewitt 2012: 4).

Roz is interested in the 'subjective experience' of women of humanistic-integrative therapy, after having been diagnosed on the schizophrenia/schizo-
affective disorder (S/S-AD) spectrum. The dual focus on subjective experiences
and humanistic-integrative therapy is, asserts Roz, underrepresented in
research today. She asserts that: 'Scientific research into the subjective experience of [Humanistic-integrative (H-I) counselling/psychotherapy] ... appears to
be virtually non-existent' (D'Ombraine Hewitt 2012: 4) and she uses this as a
trigger for further research. The overarching aim for Roz's study is, in this
sense, to contribute with research based on the lived experience of clients,
rather than to contribute to generalisations and official guidelines. Roz is

interested in 'the subjective experience of H-I therapy and its impact on the recovery of eight women with a diagnosis of S/S-AD'. She chose the Interpretative Phenomenological Analysis (IPA) as her approach to reflect the 'dynamic, subjective nature of psychotherapy' (D'Ombraine Hewitt 2012: 4).

A final example of a research problem is chosen from a different interest area and a study guided by a heuristic rather than phenomenological approach: 'Exploring the use of clay as therapy: Towards a formulation of a theoretical model' was a research project undertaken by Lynne Souter-Andersson.

Case study

Lynne Souter-Andersson (2011) refers to her research questions and objectives as follows:

> This study explores the use of clay in therapy. It records clay being used in a variety of settings and evaluates – through a series of adult research workshops, how clay is used in therapy by analysing what takes place between the client, the therapist, and the clay. The emerging strands were investigated to see if it was possible to formulate a theoretical underpinning for clay use in therapy...
>
> When clay is used in therapy what happens? How does it happen, and is it feasible to formulate a theory to underpin the use of clay in therapy?
>
> The objectives ... were many:

- To publish a book which described therapeutic work with clay that has taken place within Western Europe, but with international clients, trainees and psychotherapists.
- To illuminate present therapeutic practices using clay as a medium through the writing up of case studies.
- To describe the practicalities of using clay in a therapeutic space.
- To anchor the use of clay theoretically as a medium in its own right.
- To explain what makes clay powerful as a medium in therapy and its links with neurobiology and embodied knowing.
- To record contemporary training workshops using clay therapeutically.
- To offer ways of working in clay with adults individually or as couples, adolescents and children in therapeutic sessions.
- To explain the benefits for working with clay therapeutically for those displaying diverse needs such as small children, mental illness sufferers, disabled clients, self-elected mute clients, the elderly and those where English is a second language.

> All objectives have been met and developed further as the research got underway, leading the work into unknown and unrecorded areas; the theory-building phase of this project provides an example of this.

Again, the background for Lynne's interest in this research involves many strands. It is clear that it has taken time and effort to narrow down the focus of the research question(s) above. In the case study below, Lynne describes her 'early interest in the use of clay in therapy'.

Case study

An early interest in researching the use of clay dates back to 1988 when I was teaching in a Cambridgeshire Community Village College. I recall parent consultation evenings when I explained how there were few failures experienced when working with clay in the pottery lesson. Most students left the lesson with a sense of achievement because they had been able to produce a creation they liked or had perhaps just experienced the pleasure of playing with clay. This was certainly pre-National Curriculum Level days! A year later I began psychodynamic training to become a counsellor. ... Clay seemed to have a way of touching that which sought to be touched and worked through. ... Whilst I have over three decades of experience teaching art and pottery to secondary aged youngsters in England, which has contributed significantly in understanding how youths responded to clay in an educational setting, I wanted to consider carefully how best to collate a body of knowledge that would support the use of clay in therapy sessions. In other words, how could I combine my many years of teaching pottery, plus working with individual clients using clay and the training I delivered, to present to the therapy world a body of knowledge that could provide a theoretical base for underpinning the use of clay in therapy? Mindful of Moustakas' advice, I stated the research question in 'simple, clear and concrete terms' (1990: 41). ... The structure of this comprehensive arts-based and practice-based heuristic study comprised five research components. Research component one was a gathering of previously written testimonies covering the therapeutic use of clay in non-therapy environments. The second component reviewed therapeutic professionals' experiences when clay has been used. Interviews with ten studio potters were designed as the third research component. The fourth component involved one hundred participants in clay research workshops where an analysis of the written responses to three clay exercises was studied, to see what the story of the emerging data illuminated. Finally, the fifth component was a bridging process between data collection and data analysis, since this process relied on immersion into the explicated aspects of theoretical concepts emerging from the previous four components. The intention here was to support a possible formulation of a theoretical underpinning for the use of clay in therapy.

Activity

At this stage it might be helpful to return to your earlier notes about research interests. Use what you already have formulated as potential topics, or add to the list whatever new ideas you may have come up while reading about Melanie, Roz and Lynne.

Consider your topic(s) with Dawson's (2009: 6) 'five Ws' in mind.

- **What?** Sum up you research in one sentence only.
- **Why?** Why are you interested in the topic? Is it, for instance, to improve your practice? Or maybe there is a gap in the literature?
- **Who?** Who are your participants? What type of people does your research interest involve and concern – adults, children, clients, students ...?
- **Where?** Where will your practice-based research be based – in a therapy agency, hospital, prison, school, hostel for homeless, etc. ...?
- **When?** What kind of time scale have you got in mind?

Before refining the problem, we must look into literature that is relevant to our problem. The literature review is usually an ongoing project, and can often feel like the opening of a can of worms. There is an enormous amount of research and development being published today, and Aveyard (2010: 8) describes the literature review as like bringing a jigsaw puzzle together. It is often during the research review that both the research question and the sense of methodology take shape, partly as a consequence of comparing our angle to a problem with the approaches adopted by others. Some findings will resonate and excite, while others may leave you bored, disinterested and even annoyed. Pitching one's own interest and attitude to a question against others is invaluable for narrowing down and identifying what you are precisely looking for and seeking to contribute to.

In the following chapter, Simon du Plock shares his experiences and thoughts around this important stage of research. Simon speaks from experience of being a research student as well as a head of a practice-based research programme. His additional interest in using literature in psychotherapy makes Simon ideal for writing about the merits of literature in real-life research. As Simon suggests, it is not really until we immerse ourselves into other people's research that our own research acquires its final shape.

Recommended reading

Bell, J. (2010) *Doing Your Research Project: A Guide for First-Time Researchers in Education, Health and Social Science*. Maidenhead: Open University Press.

This is a practical guide for those who want to develop their study skills.

SIX　Doing your literature review

Simon du Plock

Your literature review is a piece of research in its own right. In this chapter, Simon shares some of his experiences from this kind of research. He highlights how significant it is to engage critically with literature in order to define and refine our own research area

- Dissertation
- Problem formulation
- Literature search
- Literature research
- Synthesising
- Data evaluation
- Analysis and interpretation
- Scholarly positions
- Reflective practice
- Reflexive stance

Initial reflections

I find, as I set out on the composition of this chapter, that I am thrown instantly back into the frame of mind which occupied me when I wrote my own doctoral thesis, and that these sensations are coloured also by my memories of conducting research for two previous Master's degrees. The feelings which flood in are quite mixed, but overall they are feelings of being lost, being daunted and inadequate to the literature review task. I am surprised by the immediacy of these sensations, given that I have assessed approaching fifty doctoral dissertations (and as many Master's dissertations), and have, over the last twenty years, directly supervised dozens of doctoral candidates. Yet, upon reflection, these personal feelings should not surprise me when I recollect that they were evinced by nearly all the students with whom I have worked professionally.

Graduates of the Doctorate in Psychotherapy by Professional Studies report they had similar feelings on approaching their literature reviews. Maxine recalls:

> I felt completely overwhelmed by it and it left me feeling unsure, inadequate and fearful about where to start, how to start, and what to write. I also believed I was alone with this because I believed that everyone at doctoral level would be well acquainted with writing literature reviews and so they would know what to do and I didn't – leaving me the failure.

Claire recollected:

> To start with I was worried about the literature review. I imagined that I would have to show that I was aware of everything in the field and that it would take a very long time. Therefore the reading I did before I started writing was rudimentary and consisted of general awareness of the main writers and researchers in the area and a review of books I already owned. On reflection, because I was daunted by it, I didn't want to do it.

Clearly, there is something about undertaking a literature review which can throw us back on ourselves and make us feel de-skilled in a very particular way, even when, as in Claire's example, we are in fact engaging efficiently with the task. I find this interesting, since, in many respects, the literature review might be thought to be one of the least problematic and most tightly boundaried components of any research undertaking. Yet much rides on the creation of a competent literature review and a flawed review will throw doubt on the validity of the research which it informs: as Boote and Beile (2005: 3) state, 'a researcher cannot perform significant research without first understanding the literature in the field'. Mullins and Kiley (2002: 377) found in their research on how examiners assess doctorates that: 'The initial impressions of the quality of the thesis are usually formed by the end of the second or third chapter of the thesis – often by the end of the literature review'. Moreover:

> Examiners typically started reviewing a dissertation with the expectation that it would pass; but a poorly conceptualized or written literature review often indicated for them that the rest of the dissertation might have problems. On encountering an inadequate literature review, examiners would proceed to look at the methods of data collection, the analysis, and the conclusions more carefully. (Boote and Beile 2005: 6)

Beginning to write

Where can the student turn for support in negotiating these rapids, which are capable of fatally damaging their delicate research vehicle at such an early stage in the research journey? Boote and Beile (2005: 5) assert:

> Doctoral students seeking advice on how to improve their literature reviews will find little published guidance worth heeding. ... Most graduate students receive little or no formal training in how to analyze and synthesize the research literature in their field, and they are unlikely to find it elsewhere.

Consulting my book shelves for texts I used in my own doctoral research, I find my 1999 edition of Graves and Varma's *Working for a Doctorate* lists only six books or book chapters on writing theses. While there are still comparatively few texts devoted to this subject, a considerable body of information, much of it on the web, now exists to steer the novice through the specific process of a doctoral literature review. This resource has been developed in tandem with the expansion of higher education and there is an increasing emphasis on a requirement for students at Bachelor's as well as Master's level and beyond to demonstrate their ability to both engage with published research and to carry out their own research projects. The quality and clarity of this information is variable, with that created by universities for the guidance of their students probably the most consistently reliable. There is relatively little variation between the available advice and, consequently, the production of a literature review may be seen as a fundamentally technical exercise – one in which the artistry of the individual practitioner has only limited relevance. There is, on this reading, a 'right' way to create a literature review, or at least a series of steps the writer needs to take which, if followed correctly, will, like a trusted recipe, produce a piece of writing which can be termed a 'literature review'.

Typically, these resources define the concept of a literature review, expanding on the premise that it is an account of what has been published on a topic by accredited scholars and researchers, and stipulating what it must do. In the case of the University of Toronto website (www. writing.utoronto.ca/advise/specific-types-of-writing/literature), for example, it must:

- be organized around and related directly to the thesis or research question you are developing
- synthesize results into a summary of what is and is not known
- identify areas of controversy in the literature
- formulate questions that need further research.

The reader is given specific direction, too, on the components of a literature review: the University of California, Santa Cruz, website (www. guides.library.ucsc.edu/write-a-literature-review), for example, lays down that a literature review should be developed via four stages:

- Problem formulation – which topic or field is being examined and what are its component issues?
- Literature search – finding materials relevant to the subject being explored.

- Data evaluation – determining which literature makes a significant contribution to the understanding of the topic.
- Analysis and interpretation – discussing the findings and conclusions of pertinent literature.

This website goes on to state the elements which comprise a literature review as:

- An overview of the subject, issue or theory under consideration, along with the objectives of the literature review.
- A division of works under review into categories (e.g. those in support of a particular position, those against, and those offering alternative theses entirely).
- An explanation of how each work is similar to and how it varies from the others.
- Conclusions as to which pieces are best considered in their argument, are most convincing of their opinions, and make the greatest contribution to the understanding and development of their area of research.

Since such resources seem to be aimed at researchers in general, and offer advice which is necessarily generic, their authors pay little attention to the 'person' of the researcher, or to the role of the researcher in shaping their material. Lee (2009: 56) goes some way to put the researcher at the centre of the creation of the literature review by formulating a shortlist of questions aimed at clarifying how existing literature illuminates our professional practice. The researcher is urged to reflect on:

- Why am I reading this?
- What are the authors trying to do in this writing?
- What are the authors saying *that is relevant to what I want to find out?*
- How convincing is what the authors are saying? (This may include, but is not limited to, issues of quality that may involve *relevant* methodological flaws).
- In conclusion, what can I make of this? This is the 'so what?' question, which involves assessing a particular text given your chosen topic.

Such a mindful approach is likely to mitigate against what Kasket (2012: 69) calls 'the sin of the uncritical literature review', in which the reviewer produces a

> ...list-like description of other people's work with no attempt at critical analysis or synthesis. In its worst form one sees a paragraph on what Jones said, then the next paragraph is what Taylor said, the next is what Beck said, and so forth. (Kasket 2012: 69)

As important, it also encourages the reviewer to adopt a genuinely scholarly position in relation to earlier work, engaging with it via the lens of intellectual curiosity in order to assess its relevance to their own research topic – the difference between balanced critique and defensive criticism aimed at justifying the value of the proposed research. Such a scholarly position, if adopted seriously, is likely to lead the researcher to make valuable connections with existing authorities in their field. In the process, the researcher moves far beyond any mechanical compilation of previous work, and is taken towards a *live* literature review, in which they make direct contact with senior authors. As Maxine recalls:

> I gained the confidence through the literature review to contact the authors who had written articles. Often the email addresses are on the bottom of papers in journals and I would email and then I phoned and Skyped a couple of times. Authors were always supportive. Mick Cooper from Strathclyde University suggested I read and contact Bill Stiles in America who developed the 'problem of assimilation' model. They were really very helpful and guided me where to read next. Generally, doctoral candidates will receive a positive response because it is about building on theory.

These findings are echoed by Claire, when she writes:

> As I continued in my research, conversations with supervisors, peers, tutors and colleagues resulted in their suggesting books and papers, some were given to me. ... I was also in touch with other writers in the field and they let me know of new publications ... it seemed that once I embarked upon the research there was support from many unexpected avenues. I was alert to opportunities that were relevant and the task that at first seemed onerous proceeded organically.

Taking a reflexive stance

As *practitioner* researchers, though, we are in a position to take a more radical stance towards the literature review, one congruent with our approach to research *per se*. By this, I wish to remind us of the organising principle of reflexivity which informs both our clinical and our research activities, and which is discussed at length in this book. This reflexivity offers us a way of engaging with the *entirety* of the research journey, including, of course, the writing of the literature review. I have argued (du Plock 2010) that the notion of the neutral, objective researcher is as absurd as the notion of the neutral, objective therapist. In both cases the illumination they can provide depends upon who they are – or perhaps *where* they are – in relation to either the client or the topic of research. This point is as applicable to the creation of the literature review as it is to the rest of the research journey. I have found it helpful to conceptualise this 'whereness' (following the existential psychotherapist Rollo May's notion that asking a client where they are is more revealing than asking them how they are) in terms of 'research trajectory', by which I mean the angle at which the researcher enters into an explorative process, in this case the exploration of literature relevant to the research project. The angle at which one enters this field of inquiry determines what is illuminated, and also what is thrown into shadow. I say 'thrown into shadow' because there is neither light nor shadow prior to the advent of the inquirer. As this trajectory serves to privilege some aspects of the phenomenon (the body of existing literature) under consideration, and will obscure others, it is important for the researcher to be aware of their subjective stance at the outset of their research. But we need to take a further step since there is limited value in merely disclosing our subjective stance; to be truly reflexive we must also evidence our thinking about how this stance might impact upon our study, and, crucially, we need to say how we intend to manage this.

When we set aside the possibility of being a neutral investigator, we find we are called upon to describe as clearly as possible our own research trajectory in relation to our research topic. My view, as an existential therapist, is that I am attempting no more than to take seriously the axiom of existential-phenomenological investigation that the 'co-researcher', a term used to indicate the co-constructedness of 'reality' entailed in both therapy and research, should pay appropriate attention to the meanings they bring to the phenomenon under consideration. Ruth Behar (1996: 13), writing about 'humanistic anthropology', makes clear that researchers who locate themselves in their own texts forfeit the defensive position of 'scientific observer':

> Writing vulnerability takes as much skill, nuance, and willingness to follow through on all the ramifications of a complicated idea as does writing invulnerably and distantly. I would say it takes yet greater skill. ... To assert that one is a 'white middle-class woman' or a 'black gay man' or a 'working-class Latina'... is only interesting if one is able to draw deeper connections between one's personal experience and the subject under study. That doesn't require a full-length autobiography, but it does require a keen understanding of what aspects of the self are the most important filters through which one perceives the world and, more particularly, the topic being studied.

Activity

Take a few minutes to think about a topic on which you might wish to conduct a piece of research, or on which you are already engaged on a research journey. Note down what comes to mind in relation to the following questions:

- What is it about this particular topic which engages your attention?
- Do you have some first-hand experience of it yourself, or is it something which has come to your attention less directly? In either case, how does the way you have come to be aware of it suggest ways for discovering more about it?

- What is your 'felt-sense' of the topic? What is your emotional sense of the topic, and does this lead you to some ideas about how you might explore it?
- As you engage with this exercise, do you notice that you have any particular biases or assumptions in relation to the topic? Do you feel 'something must be done' or, alternatively, do you feel relatively dispassionate and objective about it?
- In what ways might these reflections inform how you could go about exploring existing work on your topic?

We should remember that is as important to be a reflective researcher as it is to be a reflective practitioner. With everything we read, we should attempt to develop a reflective process that records our responses effectively and meaningfully, and we should constantly critique our own processing of literature from where and how we are looking for it right through to what we have done with it as a result of that critique. The basis of this is to apply the same critical faculties to our own assessments of the literature that we find. In this way we take 'reflective practice' a step further to 'reflexive practice'. Reflexive practice requires us to reflect on each aspect of our own work just as we would with the work of others.

When reflecting on our work we can go further, however: for example, we can ask ourselves searching questions, and get detailed answers, about how we felt, what our private expectations were and whether they were fulfilled, where our allegiances *really* lie, whether we have an 'agenda' for what we would wish studies to show, and so on. We can also keep asking perhaps the most important question of all – was this useful, and if so how? Conversely, critical, reflective and reflexive practice also allows us to ask, if it was not useful, why not? Keeping a research journal can play a valuable role in ensuring that the literature review is distinctively *ours*, and does not fall into the trap of becoming a tedious catalogue of barely connected references. Regular inclusion of material from our journal will encourage us to relate an engaging story which will reveal how we approached the literature review, the choices we made for the inclusion of some material and the exclusion of other material, and the way our research question/questions surfaced in the process. It is possible to weave this reflexive material into the body of the literature review, include elements of it in 'story boxes' at relevant points in the text, or even present it as a time line running in parallel with the main text – the crucial point is that this strand within the research journey should be visible and available to the reader even if, in the last instance, it appears as a clearly signposted appendix.

Activity

With any paper you choose to read, give yourself 45–60 minutes to read it and reflect on the following items (the time will reduce as you become more skilled at reading research papers). In your journal, for any article that warrants it (including bad papers, not just good ones), write a reflective piece that incorporates:

- The reference details for the article
- A summary of the article in your own words
- What you learned from the article. How the findings of the article might inform your practice
- The methodological strengths and weaknesses of the study (i.e. what made it convincing? What undermined its credibility)
- Be sure to carefully note things to be looked up (e.g. books or papers in the reference list that look interesting, words, concepts or technical terms that were unfamiliar to you)
- Give the paper a star rating – was it worth five stars? Was it so poor in your estimation that it deserved none at all?

This sort of activity not only builds the ability to be a critical consumer of research, it is also preparation for an important scientific activity (one that many Doctoral candidates fulfil after their studies, if you don't already do so on the strength of your experience in the field to date), that of reviewing pre-publication versions of papers submitted to journals to assess their suitability for publication. If you don't already do this for journals, you will rapidly find that repeating this exercise at least once per week will give you the skills to do so and become one of the gate keepers of science itself.

Literature review as literary research

As we begin to review the literature surrounding the proposed research theme, we hopefully will begin to locate ourselves and our study within the wider academic field as well as alongside other research studies. In reading about inquiry rather than doing it, we may now begin to feel impatient to start the fieldwork itself and long for something more tangible than reading and sifting through ever more abstract information to produce an ever-expanding literature search. But it is important to stay with this review process: it is a valuable fermentation stage that sets the scene for what will follow. Besides, unless we know what has been done before, in research terms, we might be condemned to repeating history by merely replicating the shortcomings of earlier studies. In this way, reading will familiarise us with the wider field while developing expertise and specialist knowledge of our chosen research topic. Students are sometimes surprised to find that little has been published which relates directly to their own topic. As Rosalind discovered:

> ...I expected the literature review to be arduous, absorbing and spark new ideas about my topic. But as it became clear there was little research on my topic I did not have to read and evaluate numerous studies so it was relatively straightforward and not the mammoth task I'd envisaged. And the scant research encouraged me to think mine was a topic long overdue for investigation!

The relative paucity of existing material was, in this case, indicative of something significant and worthy itself of exploration:

> ...seemingly psychotherapy researchers into mental illness were predominantly uninterested in the personal experience of their participants.

Stella found the limited amount of existing material actually vindicated her in her choice of research topic:

> I began by thinking it [the literature review] was just something that had to be done but as I got involved and recognized the lack of relevant studies, it became worthwhile as it highlighted the significant need for research to be done in this neglected area.

We should remember that the research review is *not* a one-off process and will grow – and become more systematic – throughout our research journey; we will also need to refer back to this earlier reading at the analysis stage when we begin to appreciate 'whose thinking' and 'what earlier recorded themes' our research supports or challenges. Invaluable advice, if deceptively simplistic at first thought, is to note the whole reference for what we read, complete with page numbers for any quotes noted (this can save a quite remarkable amount of time when we reach the writing-up stage by avoiding retracing steps, the detail of which is, by then, long forgotten).

It is also important to bear in mind right from the outset that when we actually come to writing up the literature review chapter, it is preferable to critique and compare the contributions of others, rather than merely describe their work; in this regard, depth is more important than range. It also suggests that entering into a dialogue with the authors we read – where literature is evaluated in relation to our 'research question' – is far more valuable than simply collecting ever more information. So we should compare and contrast our literary sources and, as it were, set them in dialogue with each other. We may challenge and fall out with them, and even become passionate about some of them, but always with a sense of the critical and an acceptance that our favourite may turn out, like so many loves, to be built on sands that change with time. In this way we own our biases and support those who seem to echo our own 'lived experience'. In all of this it should by now be evident that the literature search is, in fact, 'literary research' – an inquiry in its own right and not to be skimped or hurried through.

Activity

These activities are designed to introduce reflection about reflection, what might perhaps be called 'reflection squared', and thus complete the reflective practice cycle:

- What routine tasks could you set yourself to help you develop your use of your research journal and to make the most of it?
- What other tasks could you set yourself, perhaps as a one-off developmental activity, to help you focus on each stage of your journey as a researcher?

My academic adviser kept saying 'don't split the research into separate sections – it's all one journey', and that felt confusing at first because in my Master's degree I approached it as one section, then the next, and the next... But I quickly realised it made perfect sense and the personal and professional review flowed into the literature review, and my journal ran alongside it all.

Concluding reflection

In conclusion, I think it is important to approach the creation of the literature review with the understanding that its function is not only to show the reader that you have explored relevant existing publications; it is also, and more fundamentally, the process by which the researcher identifies their specific research focus. Denise captured this when she wrote:

> There was no doubt in my mind this was my literature review. It was rigorous and you could see exactly how I had done it, but beyond that you could see what it was about me as a therapist with my training and background and specialism that informed it. Someone else would have written a different review – the underlying principles would have been different.

And Claire communicates the profound way in which the literature review can become a valuable and integral part of the overall research journey, congruent with the spirit of this journey, while providing the evidence base for it:

> I feel that the way that I worked with literature was entirely compatible with the rest of my project. Throughout I allowed myself to wander, with a sense that I was discovering a path that opened up before me as I walked. ... The literature review was an aspect of the preoccupation and absorption that my research became while I was doing it. ... A lot of what I read was left out [in writing up] but remained within me as an influence in my thinking.

It will be evident that the doctoral graduates I have quoted in the course of this chapter undertook their literature reviews from the same reflexive perspective as that with which they pursued their entire research journeys. In so doing, they were able to use it as an expression of their personal and professional development and make it central to their research projects. As Kasket (2012: 69) expresses it:

> ...[W]hen you embark on your literature review, you are not doing that with a research question. You are doing that with a research area. You are not supposed to have a specific research question at the beginning of your research process. ... The research question is only defined, refined, and discovered through the process of critical engagement with the literature.

Recommended reading

Aveyard, H. (2010) *Doing a Literature Review in Health and Social Care: A Practical Guide* (2nd edn). Maidenhead: Open University Press.

Aveyard's book is recommended to those who want to deepen their knowledge in evidence-based systematic approaches and compare it with the literature reviews that emphasise reflexivity.

SEVEN   Considering ethics

The relationship between researcher and research participants is typically close in practice-based research and needs to be carefully negotiated. This chapter sets out to explore the links and differences between research relationships and therapeutic relationships, and looks at ways to prepare for personal change and growth in both.

- Research invitations
- Consent forms
- Therapeutic relationships
- Confidentiality
- Good practice
- Ethical guidelines
- Narrative inquiry
- Personal change
- Ongoing consent

Although researchers–participants and therapists–clients enter a relationship for different reasons, it is important to plan for personal change and growth in both types of relationships. Etherington (2004) compares reflexive skills with the skills required in counselling and psychotherapy:

> Sometimes students arrive on research training courses believing they have to leave behind all the knowledge and skills they have acquired through counsellor training. They think they have to be 'academic', by which they usually mean 'intellectual', 'in my head', 'scientific'. They are often pleasantly surprised to discover that reflexive research training uses and values all that they bring with them and come to value. ... It could be argued that as counsellors/therapists we do not need to adopt a new role of 'researcher' because every encounter with our clients is itself a re-search activity. (Etherington 2004: 210)

There are, however, also some significant differences between the research and the therapeutic relationship. One major difference is, as Etherington (2004: 210) puts it, that 'as a counsellor people seek me out, as a researcher I seek them'. This has an inevitable impact on the dynamic of the relationship. Etherington (2004: 210) continues:

As a therapist my purpose is to assist my clients' re-search ... and in my role as researcher the positions are reversed: they are there to assist me in discovering something about a topic or concept that I am curious about.

The actual context is only one aspect of real-life research. Our 'attitude of mind' (Robson 2002: 10) is significant, with regard to our research environment. Rather than seeking to adopt the stance of someone neutrally observing from outside, we become part of the study. Robson quotes Hall and Hall (in Robson 2002: 11), who stress the importance of engaging in a research relationship:

> The research relationship is between equals and is not exploitative; the client organization is not being 'used' merely to develop academic theory or careers, nor is the academic community being 'used' (brains being picked). There is a genuine exchange. The research is being negotiated.

Practice-based research involves ethical guidelines which put the client's interest first. The basic requirement for any kind of practice-based research in the field of psychotherapy involves, at the very least, as McLeod (2012: 13) highlights:

- Informed consent
- Confidentiality
- Avoidance of harm

Many avoid research which involves one's own clients for ethical reasons. When therapists want to share their learning experiences with the therapeutic community, such as in the example of Yalom's experiences of counter-transference, cited in Chapter 1 (Yalom 1991), there are several ethical issues to consider. McLeod (2012: 14, my bullet points) addresses some of the issues in the list below. We need to secure that 'prospective informed consent for in-principle case study participation is

- obtained from clients before the commencement of therapy, and then at all further stages of the inquiry cycle up to and including the final release to publish (process consent).
- The person who undertakes the informed consent procedure should not be the therapist conducting the case.
- In situations where prospective informed consent is not feasible (e.g., a decision to conduct a case study made following commencement of therapy), alternative consent procedures must be approved by an appropriate institutional approval committee or board, or an equivalent consultative group, and include the involvement of an independent consultant who will undertake all negotiations with the client.
- In situations where informed consent is not possible (e.g., the client is not contactable) at least two independent expert consultants should audit all aspects of the inquiry process, as advocates of the client.'

McLeod (2012: 14) adds:

> Good practice in case study research involves providing the client with an oppor-
> tunity to comment on a draft of the case report, and to stipulate the deletion or
> disguising of material for confidentiality purposes. Good practice involves
> encouraging the client to make a personal statement about the case report, to
> be included in the final published version.

The therapeutic value for the client is always an overriding priority, which
won't change for the sake of research. A rule of thumb is thus to ask the
question 'will the client benefit in a therapeutic sense from that research
is being introduced?' The impact of a practitioner moving from being a
therapist to a researcher is highlighted in the following activity.

Activity

McLeod (2012: 15) suggests that we consider the following issues ourselves:

- Imagine that you are a client who has completed long-term therapy with a
  therapist whom you like and respect.
- This is the final review session at the end of therapy.
- Your therapist says that he/she wishes to write up your case for publication,
  and is asking for your approval.
- What are the thoughts, feelings, questions, fantasies etc. that you experience on hearing this request?

As suggested, even if the research does not include your own clients, the
ethical guidelines for psychotherapists usually remain. The case study
below illustrates how Isha (Mckenzie-Mavinga 2005: 23) reflects over the
issue of ethics.

Case study

The researcher's role as black facilitator, tutor, researcher and 'insider outsider'
played an important part both in the challenging nature of this study and as
a model for developing safety and compassion to facilitate the process. ...
Involving students in a study needed to be carefully considered. There were
concerns about consent as I was introducing workshops on my study theme into
their training with the agreement of colleagues rather than with the permission
of the students.

Ethical considerations

I initially engaged an ethical committee. I invited a colleague from Uni-one, a colleague from Uni-two and a colleague completely separate from my work with the training courses, but involved with diversity issues and BACP [British Association for Counselling and Psychotherapy] concerns. I was also thinking more methodologically and I asked them to give me reflective feedback on some issues of non-maleficence, which might help me cope with defensiveness, silences and the impact that participant responses might have on me.

It was my aim to collect data in a non-biased way and with informed consent. I was attempting to approach this from the position of my dual role of Tutor/researcher. I was aware that this duality may, particularly, affect trainees who might be concerned that their work may be assessed differently according to how they respond. Below I will present the ethical considerations that were taken into account.

1   **Intention**: [To] address some of these concerns in a letter to trainees that would accompany any questionnaires or verbal evaluation sessions. I briefed interviewees and trainees on issues of confidentiality and consent verbally before accepting their contributions.

2   **Confidentiality and informed consent**: Every individual was offered the opportunity to remain anonymous. Interviewees were given an opportunity to choose their own pseudonyms. Strict confidentiality was maintained.

  (a)   To ensure anonymity and permission for use of transcripts in publications, written consent was requested for those involved in recorded evaluations.

  (b)   Completion of questionnaires and handing in written material such as journals was taken as informed consent to participate in the study as anonymous contributors.

  (c)   I was aware that participants may be concerned about being recognised in documented representation of the research, or in the case of trainees known to me, that their academic work may be judged differently due to comments they make in the black issues workshops.

3   **Non-maleficence** (Commitment to avoiding harm): I wanted to be mindful of the power dynamics involved in research relationships and also in the relationships between tutors and trainees. I needed to be aware not to attempt to influence participants with my knowledge and prior experience. It was my intention to supportively facilitate students' varying levels of black issues awareness. The recognition that trainees were not quite ready for my approach and the need to change the focus of the study came out of this awareness.

4   **Autonomy**: Participation in data collection was voluntary, and trainees were given an opportunity to opt out, or refuse to answer questions, without risk of repercussion in course assessment process or bias to their relationship with the training programme. (See 2c, above)

(Continued)

(Continued)

5 **Benefice** (Commitment to the clients' well-being): Trainee/participants were expected to consider their learning in view of their understanding of course requirements to become competent counsellors, understanding, practising and supporting counsellor/client relationships for the benefit of the client. (In accordance with the BACP code of ethics; BACP 2007).

6 **Justice**: Trainees/participants were offered opportunities to integrate their learning into the theoretical and philosophical aspects of the training and practice seminars. They were also encouraged to develop their wisdom, knowledge and self-awareness of the phenomenon of black issues as it links to their own life experience, cultural experience and oppressions.

7 **Self-respect**: Trainees/participants were offered opportunities to process and exchange support about their learning and self-development that arose from their experiences of the phenomenon of black issues. They were also expected to address personal issues that arise from this work, in their therapy and personal development forums, including clinical supervision.

One of the issues which Isha reflects over in this case study is how to capture written 'reflective feedback' from the participants. She is particularly interested in monitoring the ambiguous power-balance between the participants and herself. Isha refers to the innate power imbalance in the research-relationship, particularly as a result of the dual roles of being both trainer *and* researcher. Aiming for 'non-maleficence', Isha shares how she hopes that reflective feedback from the participants 'might help me cope with defensiveness, silences and the impact that participant responses might have on me'.

Activity

How would you feel about being asked to participate in a research project, after enrolling on a counselling training course? List at least three concerns. How, if at all, could these issues be 'solved'? What could be done by the trainer-cum-researcher to put your mind at ease?

We have looked at clients and students, but the collaborative nature of practice-based research requires careful negotiation regardless of whom we engage with. Josselson (2011: 46) concludes that 'in order to obtain rich and meaningful material in the interview, we enter a relationship of trust, respect, and empathy with our participant – an I–Thou relationship in Buber's terms'. This kind of closeness and the collaborative nature of the research is riddled with ethical concerns. Josselson (2011: 46) continues:

> We have to hold this doubleness at all levels. The ethical problems here ensue from the fact that, in order to obtain rich and meaningful material in the interview, we enter a relationship of trust, respect, and empathy. ... We then take ourselves out of this relationship to communicate about some conceptual matter with our peers, making use of the interview material in an I–It manner.

The move from closeness to distance can come as a surprise for both the research participants and the researchers. But, as researchers, 'we retain a responsibility to protect those who inform us, even as we return to our colleagues to relate our own narrative of what we believe we have learned' (Josselson 2011: 34). Josselson (2011: 47) suggests addressing an informed consent both before and after the interviews.

> The concept of 'informed consent' is a bit oxymoronic, given that participants can, at the outset, have only the vaguest idea of what they might be consenting to. ... I suggested that we need to request informed consent both at the beginning and at the end of the interview .... This is because participants often don't know at the outset what they will tell us. If we interview well, we may often evoke disclosures that the participants were not prepared to reveal when they began to speak. Therefore, we need to ask them again if they consent to our using what they have revealed – after they have revealed it...

Josselson therefore encourages us to make a point of preparing our research participants for what will happen with their stories. This puts *reflexivity* to the forefront. Josselson (2011: 49) continues:

> [R]eflexivity becomes ethically necessary in the written account, not only in relation to our participants but also in relation to our readers. We need to say who we are as interpreters who bring our own subjectivity to the topic or people we are writing about. Interpretive authority cannot be implicit, anonymous, or veiled. We have to come out from behind the curtain and say who we are when we claim our authority.

This level of reflexive awareness includes emotional considerations. Josselson (2011: 44) suggests that 'participating in this process of sharing one's life to be written about by someone else stirs up a welter of narcissistic tensions in both the participant and the researcher'. Josselson (2011: 44) continues:

> I turned then to theories of narcissism to better understand what was going on. Heinz Kohut, the premier psychoanalytic theorist of narcissism, has what I found to be a useful explanation. When we work empathically in the interview situation to understand our participants, we may be evoking what he calls a 'mirror transference'. ... We have, indeed, aggrandized our participants by regarding them as important enough to write about – but the grandiose self is always tinged with shame.

Josselson (2011: 45) also reflects over the strong emotions that these processes evoke in the researcher. She writes about 'the mixture of dread, guilt, and shame which goes with writing about others and then encountering them afterwards'. Josselson (2011: 45) continues:

> The dread is easiest to trace. There is always the dread that I will have harmed someone, that I will be confronted with 'How could you say that about me?' I will discuss later the one time this happened to me. The guilt is more complicated. My guilt, I think, comes from my knowing that I have taken myself out of relationship with my participants (with whom, during the interview, I was in intimate relationship) in order to be in relationship with my readers. I have, in a sense, been talking about them behind their backs and doing so publicly. Where in the interview I had been responsive to them, now I am using their lives in the service of something else, for my own purposes, to show something to others. I am guilty about being an intruder and then, to some extent, a betrayer. This, too, is a part of me and is narcissistically difficult to manage. I realize I need to bear this guilt rather than to build intellectual rationalizations to quell it. My shame is the most painful of my responses. I suspect this shame is about my exhibitionism, shame that I am using these people's lives to exhibit myself, my analytical prowess, my cleverness. I am using them to advance my own career, as extensions of my own narcissism and fear to be caught, seen in this process.

Activity

- Discuss how you will approach ethical issues linked to your research interest.
- Will you have access to confidential information? If so, how will this be handled?
- Could your interviews, or observations, cause surprises and open up sensitive issues for the participants? If so, how will you make sure that this is appropriately communicated beforehand? How can you avoid discrepancy between prior information and the lived research experience?

Complex organisations

This final section involves gaining ethical consent in organisations where the interests of a 'multitude of parties' need to be taken into account.

Stella Gould is conducting a phenomenological inquiry into psychotherapy experienced by prisoners serving an indeterminate sentence for public protection. In the case study below, Stella shares some of her experiences from gaining ethical consent for her research in a prison.

Case study

Ethical Considerations for research in prison, by Stella Gould

A key ethical consideration is how to conduct psychotherapy with a client who is mandated to attend. ... identifies a 'core' contract between prisoner, therapist and prison management, plus the multitude of parties in contact with the prisoner inside the prison: custodial management, wing managers, prison officers, offender management, psychologists, psychiatrists, GPs and nurses, education, employers; a 'justice system' context comprising courts, probation service, parole boards, the prisoner's own legal team; the 'prisoner system' cluster of family, friends, associates (criminal and not), and victims; and finally the 'therapist' cluster of those who impact on the role of the therapist, such as supervisors and professional associations (ethics codes).

Within that complex situation, there are various practical ethical considerations:

1 The researcher works within The Ethical Guidelines for Researching Counselling and Psychotherapy of the British Association for Counselling and Psychotherapy, and also is compliant with Metanoia's Ethical Research Guidelines, together with the Ethical Guidelines for National Offender Management Service (NOMS).

2 Informed signed consent/permissions will be requested from participants.

3 Given the potential legal implications of client material the researcher will work to a strict confidentiality code, clearly indicating the boundaries of this at the beginning of any interview.

4 Names and identifiable details will be changed, this to include any family/victim or associate of the participant.

5 No information/details of prison establishments to be disclosed.

6 Participants would have the right to withdraw their consent at any time up to the final report.

7 In keeping with the Data Protection Act 1998 and Offender Management Act 2007, all recorded data will be stored in a lockable and secure cabinet and will be destroyed within one year following the completion of the final project.

8 The ethical implications of the study have been discussed with the Heads of Security and Operations for each of the prisons where this study will take place, together with the Head of Reducing Re-Offending, and they have all given written support for the study in support of the application made for Ethical Approval to Research across National Offender Management Service (NOMS).

Finally, within the prison environment there are circumstances when the researcher, and any psychotherapist, is under a duty to disclose information:

(Continued)

(Continued)

1 Behaviour that is against prison rules that can be adjudicated against (Section 51 of the Prison Rules 1999).
2 Undisclosed illegal acts.
3 Behaviour that is harmful to the participant such as self-harming or disclosure of intention to commit suicide.
4 Harm to others, i.e. prison staff, prisoners or external person(s).

These latter requirements can present an ethical challenge for researchers who must report accordingly, whilst knowing that the prisoner may well react by withdrawing from the study – or may be 'removed' from it by prison management.

Below, Stella shares with us the participant information sheet that she used in her research.

Example of participant information sheet

(Reproduced with kind permission by Stella Gould)

1. Study title:

A phenomenological exploration of psychotherapy experienced by prisoners serving an indeterminate sentence for public protection.

2. Invitation

You are being invited to take part in a research study. Before you decide, it is important for you to understand why the research is being done and what it will involve. Please read the following information carefully and discuss it with others if you wish. Ask me if there is anything that is not clear or if you would like more information. Take time to decide whether or not you wish to take part.

Thank you for reading this.

3. What is the purpose of this study?

It is hoped that by your participation in this study it will help psychotherapists, counsellors and other professionals working with offender behaviour at sentence planning so that IPP sentenced prisoners do not experience negative feelings and behaviour around its inclusion as part of their sentence plan target. The information that I get from this study may help both prisoner and professional to make a more informed decision at sentence plan stage. However, this cannot be guaranteed.

4. Why have I been chosen?

You have been chosen because you are currently serving an IPP sentence where psychotherapy/counselling were a target set for your sentence plan.

5. Do I have to take part?

It is up to you to decide whether or not to take part. If you do decide to take part, you will be given this information sheet to keep and be asked to sign a consent form.

5a. What happens if I change my mind?

If you decide to take part, you are still free to withdraw at any time and without giving a reason up to the point when the researcher begins her final thesis. Transcripts from interviews will be destroyed and recorded data will be erased by the researcher.

A decision to withdraw, or a decision not to take part, will not affect you being able to apply for counselling/psychotherapy at any time, and will not be documented into your prison records.

6. What will happen to me if I take part?

For this study I aim to collect information to answer the research question through the use of audio-recorded interviews that will last approximately 60 minutes. You will be asked a number of questions during the interview. You will be asked to attend for one interview; your responses will be analysed and compared to other participants in the study.

Please note: in order to ensure quality assurance and equity this study may be selected for audit by a designated member of the committee. This means that the designated member can request to see your signed consent form. However, if this does happen your signed

(Continued)

(Continued)

consent form will only be accessed by the designated auditor or member of the audit team.

7. What do I have to do?

You will be asked to participate in two semi-structured audio-recorded interviews when I will ask you questions concerning your thoughts, feelings, fears, hopes and expectations when you were informed that psychotherapy/counselling was a target for your sentence plan. The time and date of your interview will be made following consultation with you of a preferred time. All effort will be made to accommodate your preference within the prison regime and availability of a room where confidentiality can be observed.

8. What are the possible disadvantages and risks of taking part?

(a) It is possible that by taking part in the study you might feel some distress during the audio-recorded interview. If this should happen, I can arrange for you to be seen by a member of the counselling team for:

- A 1–1 counselling session
- advice on the location of the 'Samaritan' telephone for your wing
- offer referral to the prisoner 'listener' service

(b) Within the prison environment there are circumstances when the researcher is under a duty to disclose information to the authorities:

- Behaviour that is against prison rules that can be adjudicated against (section 51 of the prison rules 1999)
- Undisclosed illegal acts
- Behaviour that is harmful to the participant, such as self-harming or disclosure of intention to commit suicide
- Harm to others, i.e. prison staff, prisoners or external person(s)

9. What are the possible benefits of taking part?

By agreeing to take part in this study, you will be contributing valued information that will result in identifying key issues to be addressed when planning therapeutic intervention and training for prison-based psychotherapy and counselling and inter-professional learning:

- Provides an opportunity to give something back
- Promotes feelings of being valued
- Enables you to 'make a difference'

Your participation in this study will <u>not</u> allow for any reduction of your sentence or your minimum tariff date.

10. Will my taking part in this study be kept anonymous?

All information that is collected about you during the course of the research will be kept anonymous. Any information about you which is used will have your name and the name of this prison removed so that you cannot be recognised from it.

All of the data will be stored, analysed and reported in compliance with the Data Protection legislation of the United Kingdom. The data will be stored for no longer than 12 months after the end of the study. At the end of this time it will be destroyed.

11. Who has reviewed the study?

This study has been reviewed by: the Metanoia Institute and Middlesex University Research Ethics Committee.

12. Contact for further information

Stella Gould

Senior Psychotherapist

Head of Counselling

Based on Health Care

HMP XXX

Thank you for agreeing to take part in this study. You will be given a copy of the participant information sheet and a copy of your signed consent form to keep.

Participant identification number:

> ## Activity
>
> Professional organisations such as the British Association for Counselling and Psychotherapy (BACP), the United Kingdom Council for Psychotherapy (UKCP) or the British Psychological Society (BPS) etc. will provide a Statement of Ethical Practice containing information about the ethical guidelines for research. You are advised to contact your organisation at an early stage, before you start your research, in order to avoid any misunderstandings which could cause problems further on.
>
> Go to the home page of your professional organisation and log down their ethical guidelines for research. If you can't find it or access it, contact them and ask for further information.

The amount of detail provided in your code of ethics will, as Dawson (2009: 155) addresses, 'depend on your research, your participation and your methodological preferences'.

Recommended reading

Josselson, R. (2013) *Interviewing for Qualitative Inquiry: A Relational Approach*. New York and London: Guilford Press.

Josselson is a leading author in the field of ethics and narrative inquiry. In this book she describes how to cultivate skills for empathic listening and responding with an emphasis on the dynamics of the research relationship.

EIGHT   The researcher as a person

This chapter revisits and explores the researcher's personal responses in more depth. Using real-life examples, the chapter focuses on the idiosyncrasies in practice-based research, ranging from our individual ways of formulating research problems to the way we engage with our research participants and reflect on the outcome.

- Observations
- Interviews
- Reflection
- Reflexivity
- Intersubjectivity
- Voyeurism
- Supervision
- Transference and countertransference
- Validity
- Reliability
- Theory in use
- Theory in action
- Free association interview
- Epistemology

The first case study we will follow in this chapter is from Pamela Stewart's research into mother–infant bonding in prison. It forms a powerful example of how the research relationship is being negotiated with great sensitivity and care for the participants. The research is based on infant observation, as part of Pamela's MSc research for the Tavistock Institute. Pamela begins by explaining her research interest.

> By extending the observational method (Miller et al. 1993), I have studied several mothers living with their babies, all under 9 months old, in the setting of a prison. By observing different mothers and babies I hope to draw conclusions
>
> *(Continued)*

(Continued)

about the possible outcomes for these babies. ... The relationship with the mother is central to the future development of the infant. This paper explores relationships of mothers and babies in prison and considers how far effective mothering is possible in prison. The importance of the mother and infant relationship, the external environment and the people involved with the growing baby, are some of the considerations of infant observation. (Stewart 1998: 3, 4)

Esther Bick (1964, cited in Price and Cooper 2012: 56) is one the founders of infant observation. Bicks stressed the importance of capturing 'consecutive observation'. It is often in the small, seemingly uneventful, moments where life is lived. Infant observation involves, as Price and Cooper (2012: 56) put it, 'a shift of attention to the mundane'. Pamela (Stewart 1998: 3) continues:

Observing involved a carefully monitored understanding of the unique unit within the general prison setting and an attempt at understanding the impact of the work on me. ... The day begins at 7.45 when the cells are unlocked. Breakfast is at 8.00. As a response to a request by the women and the prison inspectors the evening meal is now served at the later time of 5.15. The women are then locked in their cells from 7.45pm until 7.45. ...

Pamela (Stewart 1998: 3) incorporates reflections over the emotional impact these impressions may have on her, the inmates and the others who work there:

Although I have never been in the prison at night, I am told that this can be a very frightening time with women screaming to each other, banging the windows and shouting. With only one prison officer on duty for each unit at night, many officers have told me they are uneasy. ... The prison visiting room is a highly emotional place. The women wait for their visits in a small room to the side of the large visitors' room. The women refer to this area as 'cunt's corner'. If the visitor does not arrive as planned, the women still must wait in this corner watching the other visits until the visiting hour is over. ... The unit has space for 13 mothers and babies up to the age of 9 months. During the course of the year approximately 70 babies are born to inmates. Many of the staff becomes attached to the mothers and babies.

As Hollway (2011: 57) argues, reflexivity can be said to have 'different accents'. The infant-observation model 'speaks' with a 'psychoanalytic accent'. It embraces a reflexive approach which we will return to in a section about 'psychosocial' research, and what Finlay and Gough (2003: 8) refer to as 'reflexivity as intersubjective reflection':

> The genre of reflexivity as intersubjective reflection has grown significantly ... and can be found across a range of phenomenological, feminist, psychoanalytical and ethnographic research. Here, researchers explore ... the situated, emergent and negotiated nature of the research encounter ... and how unconscious processes structure relations between the researcher and participant.

We will return to the different emphasis which can be found within reflexivity in a separate section in this book. The point being made here is the emphasis which Pamela pays to the emotional impact she might have on her research participants. She aims to avoid both 'over-involvement' and being a 'voyeuristic bystander'. She explores her role as being akin to a grandparent, who is able to 'keeping in mind events and names' and may provide a 'sense of containment for mothers and staff'.

My aim was to be a responsive presence by trying not to change what I was observing though over-involvement. I tried to hold on an 'active/passive axis' ... alive to but not dominating the frame – to stand by the women and not be a voyeuristic bystander...

... With their lacking a third party – a partner, grandparent, family member with whom to share the baby – my ability to recall past events proved meaningful. This was particularly the case when the women talked about mothers and babies who had left. Often with no photographs of their babies, the women walked a road without landmarks. Keeping in mind events and names provided a sense of containment for mothers and staff...

I participated in that I did, within the observational model, what I was asked to do. There were times, particularly at lunch, when the mothers would leave me in the nursery where I sat with 3, 4, sometimes 5 babies so the mothers could go and eat. By holding the babies, figuratively the mothers seemed held; they were able to attend to their own needs. If a baby became distressed I alerted the mother. Usually the babies sat and played...

Not all of the mothers made contact with me. Many I never got to know. I wondered about the mothers who did select me. Here no pattern emerged; some were white, some black; some foreign; some older; some younger; one a very young teenage mother. Once we had made contact the mothers would be in the nursery room waiting for me – often with their babies' dummies in their mouths. (Stewart 1998: 4)

The infant-observation model assumes that neither the researcher nor the participant escapes emotional responses to the situation and their emergent relationship. Just being in a room with others evokes all kinds of emotions. The activity below invites you to linger with the idea of you entering a room with people and to consider yourself from the outside.

Activity

Dorothea Brande, who coined the concept of 'creative writing' in the 1930s, explores writing as a way of turning ourselves and our experiences into objects of attention. This activity is actually a non-writing exercise. It is intended to be what Brande calls 'a primer lesson in considering oneself objectively'.

- You are encouraged to put any professional expectations aside, and focus on simply being you, as the one you are sitting 'with', or in, at this moment. It can be helpful to close your eyes for a moment, and concentrate on yourself – beyond roles and expectations.

Brande (1934/1996: 55) writes:

> You are near a door ... put the book aside, get up, and go through that door. From the moment you stand on the threshold turn yourself into your own object of attention.

- What do you look like, standing there?
- How do you walk?
- What, if you knew nothing about yourself, could be gathered of you, your character, your background, your purpose just there at just that minute?
- If there are people in the room whom you must greet, how do you greet them? How do your attitudes to them vary? Do you give any overt sign that you are fonder of one, or more aware of one, than the rest?

What do you feel now? Try to capture your overriding thoughts and emotions in one or two words. How do you experience yourself with others, and what that is like: positive, negative, exciting, disheartening, etc.?

A significant aspect of reflexive practice-based research is the ongoing attempt to look at problems from different perspectives and 'lenses'. Supervision is a familiar point of feedback for all therapists. The traditional use of a supervisor in research revolves around academic issues. In practice-based research, where reflexivity plays a part, the supervision tends to include support which comes closer to the supervisory experience in clinical practice. Enactments, defensive functions, over-identification, etc. are aspects which are increasingly being addressed in research-related supervision, particularly in infant observation. Both individual and group supervision are significant aspects of the actual research process because psychoanalytic researchers who 'enter the field' expect, as Price and Cooper (2012: 64) put it, to become 'exposed to primitive and unprocessed psychic material'. There is no uncontaminated position for the researcher engaged in research about emotional responses and relationships. Price and Cooper (2012: 64) continue:

> The researcher becomes a transference object for those inhabiting the field, as they do for her, and contributes to and alters the functioning of the field (even marginally)

as she becomes entangled in transference-countertransference dynamics and enactments. ... Researchers will need the help of others who are not so emotionally identified with the material in order to rediscover reflective thinking capacity in relation to the unprocessed, unconscious aspects of the material.

In the example below, Pamela (Stewart 1998: 35) shares how she feels 'scooped out and raw', and reflects over the importance of supervision to 'balance ... the very strong feelings of love and concern' which she developed:

> Over the last two years, observation became my work. The essential supervisions took the form of work discussion. I found observing enormously difficult. ... The effect on me in general was to leave prison feeling absolutely scooped out and raw. Noise hurt. I craved silence and privacy in a way that the inmates often described their experience. The sense of futility, of cycles endlessly spiralling unchecked from far back into the past and way beyond sight into the future cured me of a desire to intervene. I felt as if I was watching, perversely, an act of God unfold which no one person could stop or even stall. Action felt impossible alone. This was hard to balance with the very strong feelings of love and concern that I developed for many of the mothers and babies. In order to observe clearly I had to accept that I could do nothing more than that. Supervision was essential. Supervision evolved, taking on the quality of a work discussion. The setting was always part of the experience.

Scaife (2001: 60) asserts that strong feelings will inevitably be evoked during our kind of work and that 'the task of the therapist is not to deny them, but rather to make meaning of them in order to most usefully employ them in the service of the client'. The same perspective can be applied in practice-based research.

Validity and reliability

Validity and reliability refer to the degree to which the research can be replicated. However, practice-based research comes with all the usual 'methodological horrors' (Parker et al. 1994: 10–13) in terms of its 'indexicality', in the sense that 'all meanings will change as the occasion changes', 'inconcludability', with 'the problem that another account can add', as well as subjectivity, or the fact that 'the way we explore a problem will affect the explanation we give'. Validity involves what Parker et al. (1994: 11) describe as 'specificity rather than *replicability*':

> It is certainly possible to repeat the work that has been described, but that repetition will necessarily also be a different piece of work: different at the very least by virtue of the change of the researcher, informants and meanings of the research tool over time. The meaning that is produced in the course of research is something that has to be followed and recorded carefully and sensitively.

For research to include, rather than exclude, the complexity of the 'real', the traditional meaning of objectivity needs to be reassessed. Parker et al. (1994: 11) write:

We arrive at the closest we can get to an objective account of the phenomenon in question through an exploration of the ways in which the subjectivity of the researcher has structured the way it is defined in the first place. ... [R]esearch is always carried out from a particular standpoint, and the pretence to neutrality in many quantitative studies in psychology is disingenuous. It is always worth considering ... the 'position' of the researcher, both with reference to the definition of the problem to be studied and with regard to the way the researcher interacts with the material.

Alvesson and Skoldberg (2000: 9) contend that 'there is no such thing as unmediated results of interpretation'. Research, continues Alvesson (2002: 8), is a process of interpretation rather than a representation of reality. Alvesson illustrates his thinking with the models shown in Figures 8.1 and 8.2.

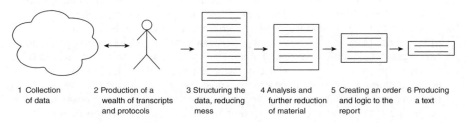

| 1 Collection of data | 2 Production of a wealth of transcripts and protocols | 3 Structuring the data, reducing mess | 4 Analysis and further reduction of material | 5 Creating an order and logic to the report | 6 Producing a text |

Figure 8.1 A simplified version of the research process, borrowed with permission from Alvesson (2002)

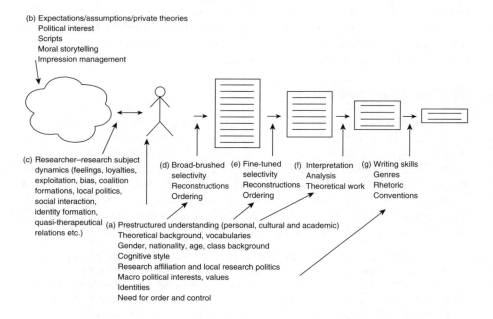

Figure 8.2 A complex version of the research process, borrowed with permission from Alvesson (2002)

Activity

Return to your earlier musings over your research interest and consider this topic in the context of your own 'subjectivity'. How might your gender, social position, early relationships, ethnicity, sexual orientation, ability, age, ethics, cognitive and theoretical constructions influence what you would like to research?

In the second main case study in this chapter, Anne Atkinson shares an example of how subjectivity impacts research, through her study in the field of 'abortion therapy'. Anne undertook her research with psychoanalytical theory as her espoused theory. She is also a Christian. Although being Christian was an aspect which Anne had been upfront with from the beginning of her research, it was something that she had expected to bracket off from her research more easily than turned out to be the case. This is something which her dialectical research process prompted her to re-evaluate. Anne chose an approach to her interviews that is called 'free association narrative interview'. The extracts below are taken from her doctoral dissertation (Atkinson 2010).

When I set out to start a professional doctorate, I had already worked on and off in the field of crisis pregnancy counselling for over twenty years. During that time it seemed evident that provision of psychological services post-abortion was negligent and that relatively few people accessed this limited service. ... I knew that I wanted my research to reflect the mind-set I inhabit in my professional life and work, desiring that the research sought to inquire beneath the words spoken in an interview, looking at what was unspoken as well as spoken in a bid to make meaning out of each participant's story. The free association narrative interview (Hollway and Jefferson 2000) fitted the bill perfectly, not least because of the guiding principle of psychoanalytic work being the free association of the mind to allow exploration without conscious censorship. I hoped that the nature of the interview might actually be therapeutic in terms of a research participant having the opportunity to tell his/her own story in a non-judgmental, reflective manner. Safeguards around not causing harm were built in to the process, with a system in place for offering help if in telling the story a participant decided that therapeutic help was indicated. I recorded the interviews and tried to transcribe these faithfully, then offering the transcript to the participant for correction and editing. There was always the opportunity to withdraw consent, and indeed, two participants did so. (Atkinson 2010: 64)

When analysing a transcript from her pilot study, Anne (Atkinson 2010: 64) reflects over how the 'transcript is borne out of a dialogue.'

> [The] the end product is not a pronounced 'truth', but a reflection of a mutual construction and one that is, in some respects, as much about me as about Lucy. ... There was the overall context of the free association narrative interview (Hollway and Jefferson 2000), so I did not introduce the interview with a question or set of questions, but merely invited Lucy to talk about her post-abortion experience.

However, Anne (Atkinson 2010: 66) engages with the transcribed interviews with a critical eye on her own input, and concludes that:

> [T]the interview itself bore the hall marks of my own self and my professional background as someone who trained as a psychoanalytic psychotherapist, and that the story that emerged would almost certainly have been told differently, and interpreted in other ways, if Lucy had been interviewed by a therapist coming from a different background.

Anne provides transcripts in her research document, and below is an extract from one of the transcribed interviews, which illustrates her point:

> Lucy: I have a couple of close friends who knew about it and that was the reason I went to Bristol: they had come from there and were going back. As much as it broke my heart, I was the one who went onto the internet and who rang and made the appointment ...
>
> Me: What was it that made you want to continue with the pregnancy?
>
> Lucy: I don't think it was anything like ... My own opinion of abortion is if it's right at the time, I'm not against it, I just believe that everybody should make their own choice and that's their decision. It wasn't because I thought I was killing a baby or any of those things, it's because if I was to have a baby, what I would do for that baby that I didn't get.
>
> Me: So the baby was really you: a tiny, vulnerable, needy part of you that you could care for.
>
> Lucy: Yes. I'm basically saying that I would give my child everything I didn't have and that's all I've ever wanted to do. It wasn't any issues like

it's bad or it's wrong or immoral. None of that meant anything to me because that's not the way I think.

Me: More like killing a part of yourself? What had been the kind of teaching you had received around it, though.

Lucy: I'd certainly never heard anything in school. There was no family opinion on it, no staunch for it or against it.

Me: *What about your religion?*

Lucy: We're members of the Methodist church. My mum attends church. I don't. My Dad didn't attend church.

Me: *So it wasn't a religious, moralistic issue?*

Lucy: No. I certainly knew of people who'd had an abortion in the past and I didn't think anything of it. (Atkinson 2010: 48)

In her analysis, Atkinson (2010: 65) explores the outcome and reflects over her own input and concludes that 'within the scope of the free association narrative interview, there is considerable leeway for influencing the way in which the story unfolds':

[When] Lucy said she wanted to continue her pregnancy because in her own words 'what I would do for that baby that I didn't get', I interpreted this as relating to her internalised fragile baby self that had never felt properly nurtured, and responded 'So the baby was really you: a tiny, vulnerable, needy part of you...' – again, using my analytic background to think about projective processes and how we use projection to deal with unprocessed internalised trauma. ... Lucy was continuing to repeat the same words whilst I spoke, and my coming in quickly with asking about the teaching she had received around abortion ... shows that within the scope of the free association narrative interview, there is considerable leeway for influencing the way in which the story unfolds, even in the absence of formalised questions ... be it real-world research or therapy.

Activity

Abortion is a sensitive subject and difficult to approach without preconceived ideas, be it that we are pro or anti, or, like Anne, are tempted to structure our hearing from a particular therapeutic model. How might your framing(s) of abortion impact the way you relate to the experience, as a researcher or as a therapist?

This research offered new perspectives on therapy linked to abortion. Anne's own experiences of how biases easily seep into the discourse about abortion would eventually influence the overall outcome of her research in terms of recommendations for art-based therapy, with as much space as possible being given to clients to create their own narrative meaning of abortion. Anne reflects:

> It seems odd to me now that I felt that I could stand apart from a client, and equally from a research participant, and somehow take a totally objective view of her/his situation, as if my own responses within an interview would not colour the very nature of the communication to some extent, and the way in which I heard and then thought about the material shared would somehow be magically separate from myself...

Reflexivity and new framings

Reflexivity involves an openness for this dynamic, and it invites us to actively engage, as Carter and Gradin (2001: 4–5) put it, 'long enough' with other world views:

> Reflexivity ... involves a back-and-forth interplay of opposing ideas [so] that differing assumptions, representations, ways of seeing, and ideas are pitted against each other. This kind of engagement leads to an understanding of opposing points of view without losing our own. ... Reflexivity, then, involves trying on the perspective, the world view of an 'other' for long enough to look back critically at ourselves, our ideas, our assumptions, our values.

This is incorporated into Anne's research after her pilot interview and further reading:

> Part of my reflexive research was to recognise how blinkered my understanding of the issue was when I chose my research topic. With regard to considering where I stood on the issue of abortion, I had to challenge my original belief that I was without effective prejudice – able to stand back and let a client decide for herself where she stood in relation to her own experience. I was unwilling to admit to myself the impact of my Christian beliefs. I told myself that I was non-judgmental and that my views would not impact on any client. I did not own the part of me that actually believed it would be better for a client to have not chosen to have an abortion, whatever the circumstances of the individual case. I began my research with an implicit, unstated assumption that any suffering post-abortion was largely consequent upon the decision made to go against the sanctity of life decreed by the Christian God. ... It was shameful to admit that I

could barely understand the value of the canter through different philosophical approaches that formed part of the early work on research methodology. As part of the research I seeped myself in the richness of the diverse models – finally recognising the value of this work – and began to evaluate and challenge the tacit knowledge that had formed the bedrock of the way I saw the world.

Anne's transformative learning illustrates, quite literally, some of the complexity involved in our attempts to 'practice as we preach'. Reflective practice invites, as in the case of Anne's study above, the researcher to move 'beyond mere description' to an analysis of 'hidden processes, decision paths and power relations in the work place', as Costley et al. (2010: 117–18) put it. The 'hidden' agendas are assumed to be found on different levels, both outside and within the researcher him/herself. Reflective practice theory is often referred to in practice-based research as capturing that ongoing 'transformational process' (du Plock 2010). Costley et al. (2010: 117–18) even muse over reflective practice in terms of a practice-based epistemology, i.e. a theory about how knowledge is being generated and construed:

> Constructing reflective practice as an epistemology ... opens up the possibility of exploring practice from a variety of perspectives. ... For the work based researcher [reflective practice] is a powerful tool for uncovering otherwise hidden processes, decision paths and power relations in the work place. It helps the researcher move beyond mere description to analysis. ... [T]he notion of the reflective practitioner ... provides a conceptual framework within which the complexities, tensions and contradictions of work can be explored, and at the same time a reference point against which the intrinsic value and practice can be judged.

Schön (1983: 49) reminds us that 'one's expertise is a way of looking at something which once was constructed and may be reconstructed at any time'. This is captured, finally, in Anne's reflections about how 'truth' really is something which is 'constructed in dialogue between individuals', and how it really did come to life during her own research experience:

> Truth began to take on a more malleable quality when viewed from kaleidoscopic perspectives. I began to embrace the realisation that even the most empirically based positivist approach was open to bias and interpretation. It was a mutative moment in the Research Challenges module [module about research methods] to take on board the idea that even at a sub-atomic level there is an intracellular effect produced by the observer. In the realm of real world research, infinite shifts in perspective and bias are integral to the way in which 'truth' is constructed in

(Continued)

(Continued)

the dialogue between individuals. This construction is a moveable feast, almost certainly subtly or overtly different according to those involved (plus a myriad of other factors), including the conditions under which the conversation/interview took place, how the individuals were feeling about themselves and each other at the time of their exchange, plus a host of environmental, religious, cultural, philosophical, psychological and physiological dimensions – to name just some of the prevailing influences. (Atkinson 2010: 11)

Countertransference in research

As researchers, we will, as Price and Cooper (2012: 64) put it, 'almost inevitably identify with research subjects and their ordinary defensive functioning'.

Although the idea of countertransference in research is usually explored in context of a psychoanalytic framework, it is worth noting that we will find this stance to research among therapists from other modalities. We looked earlier at Yalom's reference to transference and countertransference. Maxine Daniels' work (2011) is another example of a humanistic therapist who addresses the relevance of countertransference in research. We will begin with an extract from Maxine's attempt to put her choice of method into a context of her research interests. Maxine's research aim is to evaluate a role-play programme for sex offenders in prison for 'victim empathy'. Maxine (Daniels 2011: 82) explains below how her interest in 'idiographic' aspects involves a focus on the unique and the individual:

> I deliberately chose a phenomenological method to elicit the 'experience' of prisoners when undertaking victim-empathy role plays ... Smith (2004) developed a method of combining phenomenology and psychology in order to give a structure in which to examine the phenomenological data, and named it interpretive phenomenological analysis (IPA). This methodology also acknowledges the relationship between researcher and participant, in that there is always an interpretation on the part of researcher. ... The process is idiographic in nature in that it is concerned with the particular; in other words, the detail of one individual's experience, as opposed to a group of people (nomothetic) in a given context.

We will attend to the issue of methodology in more depth later on. Methodology is, as Robson (2002: 549) says, 'the theoretical, political and philosophical backgrounds to social research'. In the extract above, Maxine explains how her choice of methodology has been guided by her interest in 'capturing the quality and texture of individuals' experiences' (Daniels 2011: 83). She explains how she explored different alternatives within the family of phenomenological methods, for instance grounded theory, thematic analysis and narrative analysis. Maxine (Daniels 2011: 83) explains, further, how her chosen method, Interpretive phenomenological analysis (IPA), is used in her analysis of the data – i.e. the lengthy interviews:

> IPA uses semi-structured interviews, with questions being open ended and non-directive, and the data is analysed by the researcher engaging in an interpretative relationship with the transcript. The process is repetitive and researchers repeat the process reading and analysing the data until the themes are clustered and then finally drawn together under the super ordinate headings, or major themes. The writing up of these themes is still part of the interpretive stage, which is identified ... as having two levels: (a) a more descriptive, empathic level to allow the researcher to enter the participant's world and (b) another level of interpretation that takes it beyond the participant's own words.

Like Pamela Stewart earlier, Maxine stresses the value of supervision, which allows her the space to elicit emotional material. She describes initially that supervision always has been a natural part of her clinical practice, but how she felt unprepared for similar needs as a researcher:

> As a conscientious clinician, I know how to be non-judgmental, empathic and supportive to offenders in helping them to disclose information and work through the difficult aspects of their lives. However, I am also human, experiencing conflicting emotions that I will take to supervision in order to make sense of it by exploring the countertransference .... Strangely, I did not do this after the interviews because I was in a new role of researcher and did not equate this being a clinician and needing to seek personal support. (Daniels 2011: 62)

After interviewing the ex-offenders, Maxine transcribed the interviews. However, during the reading she noticed how she became increasingly affected by the readings. She began to put off reading certain transcripts, as described in the extract below:

> Although I have many years clinical experience working with this client group, I was not prepared in my role as researcher for the disturbing and vulnerable feelings that were evoked in me when I analysed the data. ... My first interview involved a man who had abused his daughter from the age of twelve years, continuing through her leaving home and going to university. ... I struggled at the parts where he said it was like 'having a love affair' ... reading his account line by line, immersing myself in his experience, left me on an emotional roller coaster. ... I avoided the analysis ... and would make excuses and do something else. ... I would look at my own children, especially my sixteen year old daughter, and think about how this could happen. ... I knew I had to find specific supervision. ... I also wanted someone who was a trained therapist, as I realised this material was no doubt triggering my own issues, and in order to be clear about what belonged to me and what belonged to the offender, I wanted a professional who could help me explore my own personal material. ... It was this latter area that made me realise the importance of reflexivity. (Daniels 2011: 69)

As often in the case of countertransference, the links are not always obvious. Daniels was used to working in prison and experienced in working with sex offenders. She describes how personal the link was for her, and how important it was to be able to explore the connection with a mind open for surprises:

> [The supervisor was] a counsellor who had worked in ... prison and had trained sex-offender treatment work. [In a session] my anger and tears about the injustice of this twelve-year-old had indeed resonated with me. It was about me as a young child feeling a victim, not in a sexual sense, but more in that my father died when I was five years old and the feelings of loss of power I had, and that my mother struggled to cope. It was very insightful gaining this knowledge, and feeling I was also regaining control, the separation between myself and the twelve-year-old victim helped me to process my information and then the interview. (Daniels 2011: 69)

Our own reactions will almost certainly seep into the research process at different stages of the research. As Daniels writes, supervision became an invaluable resource to help her 'to be clear about what belonged to me and what belonged to the offender'.

Activity

This exercise is about your life story.

- Return to the uninterrupted writing about 'your sock', or choose another significant personal memory to write about for five minutes.
- Now write something brief about your approach to your work. Write about your focus and special interest in work as the thoughts come into your head.

Compare the two stories. Are there any overlaps or differences? If possible, show and discuss the texts in pairs.

Recommended reading

Hollway, W. and Jefferson, T. (2012) *Doing Qualitative Research Differently* (2nd edn). London: Sage.

This is an updated version of what has become a classic within psychosocial research.

NINE Epistemology and methodology

This chapter explores the issue of epistemological positioning in our research, in particular the difference between realism, idealism and postmodern critique. It focuses on different approaches or subjectivity and objectivity in research.

- Research purpose
- Efficacy research
- Effectiveness
- Epistemology
- Realism
- Idealism
- Cartesian doubt
- The unconscious
- Lived experience
- Phenomenon
- *Noema*
- Schizoid attitude in research
- Phenomenology
- Narrative inquiry
- Hermeneutics
- Ethnography
- Constructivism
- Social constructionism
- Postmodernism
- Feminist research approach

Therapists with an interest in exploring therapeutic practice have, of course, multiple overarching choices at hand. Barkham et al. (2010: 24) suggest that we think in terms of four types of research 'to describe the domains of activity that are needed in order to provide a comprehensive approach to the accumulation of evidence'.

- Efficacy research is interested in specific, measurable aspects of treatment. It focuses on the effects of particular interventions with an interest in questions of 'safety, feasibility, side effects and appropriate dose level' (Barkham et al. 2010: 23)
- Effectiveness research often explores the efficacy research in a wider context, and explores if the isolated treatment effects can have a 'measurable, beneficial effect when implemented across broad populations and in other service settings' (Barkham et al. 2010: 23)
- Practice research focuses on variations in care and human processes rather than seeking to isolate or generalise effects of interventions. Compared to evidence-based approaches which rest on the principle that the potential for bias can be reduced through controlled experiments, the practice-based approach aims to capture and include differences and idiosyncrasies of everyday life. It aims to capture 'treatments' with reference to both the individual therapist and the clients' varying characteristics in terms of gender, ethnicity, social class as well as intrapersonal differences. Barkham et al. (2010: 39) assert that 'rather than controlling variables as in an RCT, [practice-based studies] aim to capture data from routine practice ... to reflect everyday clinical practice'.
- Service system research focuses on 'large-scale organizational, financial and policy question' (Barkham et al. 2010: 24) with delivery and optimal accessibility in mind.

Practice-based research, guided by a reflexive approach, requires sensitivity on many levels. We looked earlier at Pamela Stewart's attention to her surroundings, and at Maxine's and Anne's critical explorations of their interpretive frameworks. Practice-based research often includes differences and idiosyncrasies of everyday life, and we will look at different attempts to position the research in a personal, cultural, theoretical and linguistic context to give these kinds of studies validity with regard to the impact of subjectivity in the studies. An underlying assumption in reflexivity is that we 'arrive as close to an objective account as we can [through] an exploration of the ways in which the subjectivity of the researcher has structured the way it is defined in the first place' (Parker et al., 1994: 13).

Epistemology

Epistemology is one of the oldest branches of philosophy, and something which creates a threshold to all forms of research. Epistemology is, admittedly, as Slevin (2001: 144) puts it, 'one of those words that puts almost everyone off', yet it is 'vitally important':

> Epistemology is one of those words that puts almost everyone off. Most people cannot even pronounce it ... However, it is vitally important for all that... It is the

study of what knowledge is, how we come to know, and the nature and forms that knowledge takes. It deals with the matter of justification, the arguments we can present to justify the belief that the knowledge is in some way true or accurate. And it deals also with how we accumulate knowledge, and how we classify this knowledge. (Slevin 2001: 144)

Costley et al. (2010: 55) remind us that 'the epistemological claims you want to make from the research, the appropriateness of the methods to enable such claims, and the willingness of the community to subject itself to the methodologies, all influence the validity of the research itself'.

The validity of our research is, in this sense, linked to how we relate to and explain our understanding of 'what knowledge is, how we come to know, and the nature and forms that knowledge takes' (Slevin 2001: 144).

Realism and idealism

One significant and overarching distinction between approaches to reality is often made in terms of 'realism' versus 'idealism'. Realism implies a world view where material objects can exist independently of our senses or perceptions. This is reflected in the kind of knowledge we claim to contribute. In its strictest sense, within psychological research realism implies, for instance, that our own mind can be reduced to matter, and that mind equals the brain. Idealism, on the other hand, argues that nothing exists independently of our consciousness and our mind. Idealism is often discussed as an anti-realist theory of perception, with extreme views that objects are 'no more than collections of sensations appearing in minds' (Cardinal et al. 2004: 146).

The philosopher Berkley (1685–1753) is an example of an early Idealist. He took the concept to a level where physical objects only existed as long as we perceived them; when we leave a room, close our eyes, or in other ways retract our attention and perceptions from anything around us, it ceases to exist. Berkley coined the phrase 'esse est percipi' – 'to exist is to be perceived' (Warburton 2004:103).

René Descartes (1596–1650) emphasised the importance of certainties. He was a realist who believed in a reality 'out there', independent of our minds and perceptions. He was also a 'rationalist', and approached reality as something of which we could gain understanding through reason inspired by mathematics and geometry. Many researchers have since engaged with his ideas, either to argue for or against the notion of there being a reality 'out there' independently of us and our perception of it. Descartes suggested a dual understanding of people, with the mind and the body as separate entities, and he coined the phrase 'Cogito, ergo sum' – 'I think, therefore I am'. Descartes was a mathematician and philosopher who reasoned that the scientific knowledge of his time often was based on unreliable assumptions – 'mere beliefs', as he put it. He employed a 'method of doubt' to filter truth from mere belief in similar ways as mathematics built up knowledge in small steps. Descartes is relevant for research today for many reasons, one of them being the background picture he offers to evidence-based research. Like the evidence-based approaches, certainties are paramount in the rationalist branch of realism.

Ambiguity did not sit easy with Descartes. He set out to look for something permanent and captured the not-knowing as a dreaded place: 'In our sleep we share the weakness with "the madmen" to confuse dream for reality and give into uncertainties', writes Descartes (1641/2008: 23). He refers to fears of having to 'liken myself to madmen, whose brains are so damaged by the persistent vapours of melancholia that they firmly maintain they are kings when they are paupers, or say they are dressed in purple when they are naked ... or that they are pumpkins, or made of glass'.

Does this madness, frets Descartes (1641/2008: 22), not happen to us all in the sleep? 'As if I were not a man who sleeps at night, and regularly has all the same experiences whilst asleep as madmen do when awake – indeed sometimes even more improbable ones.'

Descartes (1641/2008: 24–5) undertakes the project of demolishing 'everything completely and start again right from the foundations ... to establish anything at all in the sciences that was stable and likely to last':

> I was struck by the large number of falsehoods that I had accepted as true in my childhood, and by the highly doubtful nature of the edifice that I had subsequently based on them. ... It feels as if I have fallen unexpectedly into a deep whirlpool which tumbles me around so that I can neither stand on the bottom nor swim up to the top. ... Whatever I have up till now accepted as most true I have acquired either from the sense or through the senses. ... [Am I really here] sitting by the fire, wearing a winter dressing-gown holding this piece of paper in my hands? ... So serious are the doubts into which I have been thrown as a result of yesterday's meditation that I can neither put them out of my mind nor see any way of resolving them. ... I realised that it was necessary ... to demolish everything completely and start again right from the foundations if I wanted to establish anything at all in the sciences that was stable and likely to last. ... I will make an effort and once more attempt the same path which I started on yesterday. Anything which admits the slightest doubt I will set aside just as if I had found it to be wholly false, and I will process in this way until I recognise something certain.

The famous 'Cartesian doubt' involved scepticism towards everything except things which could be measured. Descartes was a mathematician. His 'method of doubt' was inspired by arithmetic and geometry, and reflects the attitude of the Enlightenment triggered by the scientific revolution of the sixteenth and seventeenth centuries. We may not be certain of much, admitted Descartes (1641/2008: 23), but what we can be certain about we must find and hold onto, and then allow those findings to become guidelines for our lives as a whole:

> Arithmetic and geometry and other subjects of this kind, which deal only with the simplest and most general things ... contain something certain and indubitable. For whether I am awake or asleep, two and three added together is five, and a square has no more than four sides. It seems impossible that such transparent truths should incur any suspicion of being false. (Descartes 1641/2008: 23)

Between these orthodox views on realism and idealism, there are many variants. We discussed the idea of positivist realism in the context of evidence-based research. The philosopher Kant (1724–1804) adopted a stance called 'transcendental idealism', and proposed that there is a reality but we cannot expect to know about it on its terms. We cannot claim to know a 'thing *per se*' (*Ding an sich*) but will have to rely on our perception of the world. Although Kant (1787/2007: 341) was an Idealist, he did not go as far as Berkley, but suggested instead:

> It must not be supposed ... that an idealist is he who denies the existence of external objects of the senses: all he does is to deny that this existence is known through immediate perceptions, and to infer that we can never, by way of any possible experience, become perfectly certain of their reality.

Kant has triggered many discussions about whether a mind-independent reality exists, and if so, how to access it. Kant emphasised the role of perceptions. He argued that there 'is no possible description of the world which can free itself from some reference to experience' (Kant 1783/2008:108). He did, on the other hand, think that our ability to perceive, which included sorting and categorising information in different ways, was something we all were born with, and which, in this sense, existed 'a priori' and regardless of our doing. Kant borrowed Plato's distinction between noumenon and phenomenon and elaborated on its meaning. He used the term 'phenomenon' to describe a person's *experience of* something, and the concept *'noema'* for 'things-in-itself'. In Kant's view, humans can make sense out of phenomena in these various ways, but we can never *directly* know the noumena, the 'things-in-themselves'. When we set out to describe the object of inquiry, i.e. the noumena, we are in fact describing the manifestation of that object, as opposed to the object itself.

Searching in feebly lit areas

Some of you who expected a hands-on, demystifying approach to research might feel disappointed at this stage. Philosophy is a peculiar landscape; it is tainted by hubris, littered by disputes and disagreements, and at the same time is capable of offering magnificent vistas mixed with nourishing, soothing places to rest. Philosophy is, as Qualley (1997: 153) puts it, 'valuable not because it can uncover The Real, but because it can create alternative ways to think about whatever reality it is we've inherited/discovered/created'.

The fact that so many people have been searching for meaning for so long, is to my mind a soothing thought. I find the enthusiastic and pig-headed claims for having found the truth about our existence tantalising; they feed into my childhood dream about a consistent reality. I can also be reminded of the disappointment, frustration and unease which conflicting or nonsensical explanations about the world can trigger. I grew up with a parent who suffered from Bipolar disorders, so ambiguity was very real in our household. Personal therapy has obviously been invaluable in coming to terms with these experiences. However, to me, philosophy offers additional means to deal with questions concerning reality and the meaning of life. Kant suggested that this kind of yearning perhaps was the only thing we could be really sure about. He referred to our tendency to seek explanations as something which might even exist regardless of our mind; as an 'a priori' condition, i.e. something universal and consistent, which is there before us. Who knows?

Regardless of the motifs for our efforts to find certainties, it is easy to get lost in the process. Corradi-Fiumara (2001: 37) asserts that:

> Some of our research attitudes could be compared to the behaviour of the proverbial drunk who looks for his keys under the lamp post, not because he has lost them there, but because that is where the light is.

She reflects over how we might benefit from moving our search into outside, well-lit areas, and dare to 'touch and feel' our way:

> And yet, anyone willing to accept this image might reply that there is no way to look for something where there is no light. Perhaps the answer could come in the form of an effort to cast any feeble light in different areas, or to search in the dark by touching and feeling. (Corradi-Fiumara 2001: 37)

In her comparison between some research methods and the misguided enlightenment of the proverbial drunk, Corriadi-Fiumara (2001: 37) addresses the lack of emotions as one of the biggest problems:

> For most 'philosophers' emotions exhibit some theoretical relevance as obstacles to the progress towards truth. Whatever else affects may be, the assumption that has prevailed is that they cloud the vision of the intellect and ultimately limit freedom.

Corriadi-Fiumara (2001: 144) is missing 'the complexity, fragility and uniqueness of our being'. It is as if philosophy refers to an almost uninhabitable reality, or as Corriadi-Fiumara (2001: 7, 144) puts it, science and philosophy revolve around an 'unliveable idealised rationality ... developed from the point of view of an identity that was never born'. Science adopts a 'schizoid attitude' (Corradi-Fiumara 2001: 25) to reality, where cognition and affect are being separated.

Not being the master of our own house

Emotions were, on the one hand, the key theme for Freud. On the other hand, he preferred to look for the 'keys' in well-lit areas. It is, nevertheless, as Cottingham (2008: 291) says, 'difficult for us to comprehend what impact Freud has had' on the way we think about the self and the mind:

> Although many of the details of Freud's theories have given rise to intense critical discussion, his ideas have irreversibly changed our ways of thinking about the self and the mind, and the full implication of that is still in the process of being assimilated.

The philosopher Ricoeur (1970: 33) also highlights the impact that both Marx and Freud have had on our understanding of reality. While 'the philosopher trained in the school of Descartes knows that things are not such as they appear', he accepts the notion of consciousness, asserts Ricoeur. Freud brought to our attention that there is not only reason to doubt things, but prompts us also to doubt consciousness itself.

Freud's (1922/2008: 296) way of supporting his science with case studies became his hallmark. With reference to a case study about a woman who involved her maid in seemingly meaningless extra work, Freud (1922/2008) addresses 'the partly hidden Self':

> A lady of nearly thirty years of age suffered from very severe obsessional symptoms. ... Every time I asked the patient 'What is the meaning of it?' or 'Why do you do it?' she had answered 'I don't know'. But one day, after I had succeeded in overcoming a great hesitation on her part, she suddenly did know, for she related the history of the obsessive act. More than ten years previously she had married a man very much older than herself, who had proved impotent on the wedding night. ... In the morning he had said angrily, 'It's enough to disgrace one in the eyes of the maid who does the beds,' and seizing a bottle of red ink which happened to be at hand, he poured it on the sheet.

Comparing 'senseless obsessive acts' with memories to 'deduce the purpose of the obsessive act from its connection with the memory' when the patients are ready to make the connection themselves involved 'transforming something unconscious into something conscious' (Freud 1922/2008: 293).

Freud (1922/2008: 296) referred to the theory about our hidden parts of self as a 'bitter blow' to 'man's craving for grandiosity'. 'Present-day psychological research ... is endeavouring to prove to the "ego" of each one of us that he is not even master of his own house, but that he must remain content with the veriest scraps of information about what is going on unconsciously in his own mind.'

The reference to none of us being 'master of his own house' appears to exclude the therapist. Freud (1922/2008: 296) regards it as 'our lot' to enlighten:

> We psychotherapists were neither the first nor the only ones to propose to mankind that they should look inwards: but it appears to be our lot to advocate it most insistently and to support it by empirical evidence which touches every man closely.

The influential scientist of our time, Karl Popper (1902–94) admitted the impact Freud had on our ideas about knowledge and reality. Popper (1957/2008: 454) concludes that both Freud and Marx 'seemed to have the effect of an intellectual ... revelations. ... [T]hose of my friends who were admirers of Marx [and] Freud were impressed by [their] apparent explanatory power. These theories appeared to be able to explain practically everything that happened within the fields to which they referred.'

Popper described, however, Freud's psychoanalytic theory as 'pseudoscience'. He used Freud and Marx as examples of irrefutable observations, where truth appears manifest and impossible to prove wrong. Not being able to falsify their theories, doubting became synonymous with not *wanting* to see the manifest truth 'either because it was against their class interests or because of their repressions which were still "unanalysed" and crying aloud for treatment' (1957/2008: 454). Popper asserts:

> Once your eyes were thus opened you saw confirming instances everywhere: the world was full of verification of the theory. Whatever happened always confirmed it. ... It is easy to obtain confirmation, or verifications, for nearly every theory – if we look for confirmations. (1957/2008: 454)

Science, asserts Popper, must be based in refutable propositions; it should be based on ideas which can be tested objectively and in detached ways, ideally with doubt and suspicion as the starting point:

> Confirmations should count only if they are risky predictions; that is to say, if, unenlightened by the theory, we should have expected an event which was incompatible with the theory ... Every genuine test of a theory is an attempt to falsify it. (1957/2008: 454)

The search for certainties prevailed and was certainly adopted by Freud. He positioned psychotherapy within a deterministic model, and aimed to find a home for psychotherapy in the family of the natural sciences. It is, however, as shown by Popper earlier, not difficult to find weaknesses in Freud's claims of contributing with measurable certainties. Spence (1989: 209) highlights how the psychoanalytic model differs from the mainstream scientific tradition:

Freud insisted that the psychoanalytic enterprise has the status of a natural science. ... When we turn from how psychoanalysis is defined to the way it is reported, its scientific status becomes somewhat harder to recognise. ... [D]ata are largely private and not accessible to the curious scholar who wants to see for himself. ... [T]he privacy of the patient leads to the dubious tradition of protection through disguise. ... [T]here is no precedent for the kind of open discussion or conflicting finding that is central to the traditional scientific approach.

Freud has revolutionised clinical practice, and his impact on theory about the mind is huge, as Cottingham (2008) addressed. However, Freud's case studies make valuable social, cultural and psychological history in both a negative and positive sense. His sexists remarks – an aging man's ongoing interpretations about young girls' 'suppressed' sexual desires as being 'the problem' – provides us with plenty of evidence of how subjective the seemingly neutral observer was and perhaps will continue to be. The issue of power has been addressed, for instance, from post-structural, postmodern and feminist theory, and Freud has been heavily critiqued from pathologising women on the basis of his own skewed view about their role and their sexuality.

Overall, Freud adopted a pompous tone and an air of certainty in a 'shaded' area, or as Freud put it, where man no longer is the master of his own house. He engaged in this sense in an evidence-based, positive-realist debate about problems linked to people's fragile and ever-changing perception of reality, rather than about their reality as such. His field of study is linked to a mind-dependent reality, and is nearer to idealism than realism. Some argue that Freud was a 'misguided hermeneutic'. Frommer and Langenbach (2001: 50, 57) suggest that Freud was led by a 'scientific misunderstanding' of his own method, and actually 'used hermeneutic and qualitative methodology'. It is interesting to note how the theory of the unconscious is being revisited through neuroscience today, with its realist framework. We will also return to a psychoanalytically inspired model with reference to both the infant-observation model and the free association interview.

The lived experience

While evidence-based research is anchored in realism and strives to capture reality as such, hermeneutics, ethnography and phenomenology are examples of methodologies with an interest in people's perception of reality.

- **Hermeneutics** stress that 'we cannot separate ourselves from the meaning we gain: understanding always involves interpretations' (Finlay and Ballinger 2006: 261). It is often referred to as 'an art and a science of interpretation'.
- **Ethnography** derives from anthropology and focuses on 'description and interpretation of a cultural group or social system' (Finlay and Ballinger 2006: 262).

- **Phenomenology** focuses, in turn, 'on the way things appear to us through our experience or in our conscious' (Finlay and Ballinger 2006: 262). While the psychodynamic theory has had an enormous influence on our clinical practice and the therapeutic profession as a whole, phenomenology has been more congruent and applicable to actual research about perceptions and emotions.

The foundational figures in phenomenology are Husserl and Heidegger. Like Kant, Husserl (1859–1938) developed his thinking about perception about reality with reference to *'noema'* and our perception of things-in-themselves. Phenomenology took Kant's interest in experiences much further. Phenomenology brought emotions into the discussions, and Husserl spoke about feeling, remembering, judging, etc., rather than just as something cognitive, like perception. He approached people's emotions and perception of things (*noema*) with an interest in their subjective point of view. Husserl used concepts such as intentionality, *noema* and *noesis* to capture what these perceptions, feelings, thoughts and reflections could mean to each individual person. Husserl (1960/1999: 77) suggested that: 'the world, with all its Objects ... derives its whole sense and its existential status ... from me myself', which contrasts Kant's focus on universal and commonly held patterns for perception.

Activity

Both Kant and Husserl refer to the idea of a mind-dependent reality. Consider (or if possible, discuss in pairs) the extent to which your research interest relates to a reality which exists independently of our minds and perceptions of it.

Interviewing with shifting perceptions in mind

The phenomenological approach suggests that, as Langridge (2007: 4) says, 'it does not make sense to think of objects in the world as separately from subjectivity and our perception of them'. Phenomenology adopts 'an epistemological focus on experience or narrative (rather than a real world)'.

The way we make sense of experiences is, in turn, an ongoing process. This is reflected in the phenomenologically guided interviews. One horizon gives way for a new vista – or, as Moustakas puts it, one 'horizonal statement' gives birth to another. We can never exhaust the way we make sense of experiences. Moustakas (1994: 95) captures this suggestion as follows:

> Horizons are unlimited. ... A new horizon arises each time that one recedes. [T]hough we may reach a stopping point and discontinue our perception of something ... the possibility for discovery is unlimited.

Moustakas (1994) refers to 'interview guidelines' in his Husserl-inspired version of a phenomenological interview. The case study and activity below illustrate a research situation aimed to capture the participant's developing thinking and feeling about a phenomenon. After reading the case study, you will be encouraged to engage with another person – a peer, friend or colleague – to make an 'interview' of your own.

Case study

An important aspect of phenomenological research is to listen out for 'examples of horizontalisations', suggests Moustakas (1994: 125). They capture moments of an experience. Moustakas (1994: 65) writes:

> The noesis refers to the act of perceiving, feeling, thinking, remembering, or judging – all of which are embedded with meanings that are concealed and hidden from consciousness. The meanings must be recognised and drawn out.

He offers some examples of horizontalisations from Palimieri's investigation (Palimieri, cited in Moustakas 1994: 125) about 'the experience of adults abused as children'. Moustakas writes:

> The following horizonal statements are excerpted from the first fifth and last fifth of the research interview with Geraldine in which she recounts her experience of being sexually abused as a child by her father. Each horizon of the research interview adds meaning and provides an increasingly clear portrayal in which the abuse occurs, and the thoughts and feeling of the victims:

First fifth of the interview

- 'I remember the door and was standing in between the door to the living room and the kitchen and my dad approaching me very gently.'
- 'I am feeling, I can feel real tense, but yet having no control over the situation at all.'
- 'I think I was entering the kitchen from the living room and my dad came up from behind, from the living room. He was stirring in his chair before that.'
- 'And, as I walked into the living room he kinda caught me right then. And, just continue to perform that on me. Staring at me the whole time. Yeah, with him down on his knees, just staring up at me the whole time ....' [cont.]

Last fifth of the interview

- 'One word that comes to mind, shame. Feeling shame. I was shamed. My dad was shaming me. Made me feel dirty.'
- 'I mean at the time being just twelve years old, at the time when I should have been just starting to grow and learn about sexuality through my own experiences ... my own ... what I wanted to do ... not just being forced to do something. And I feel he just took that away from me ... [etc.].'

Activity

Divide, if possible, into pairs. Alternatively, find a friend willing to be interviewed about her/his experience of something – it can be anything which feels relevant to him/her at the time, such as leaving children in the nursery in the morning, stopping to fill up the car with petrol, arriving at work or college, or something like 'falling in love', giving birth, moving house. So, it should be an experience that matters at the time.

Prepare a couple of broad questions to obtain a 'rich, vital, substantive description' (Moustakas 1994: 116) of your research participant's experience of the phenomenon. You may want to use the following questions guided in your interview:

- Describe your initial experience of love (filling up the car with petrol, arriving at college ... or any other chosen theme). What dimensions, incidents and people stands out to you as connected with this experience?
- What where your thoughts?
- What bodily reactions can you think of?
- What feelings came up for you?
- How did the experience affect others?
- What changes would you connect with the experience – how has the experience affected you?
- Is there anything else significant which you connect with the experience?

This is an informal interview situation. However, if you prefer, please feel free to practise written consent before the interview. Examples of invitation letters and consent forms are included in this book. Before you start asking questions, prepare for the interview with your participant with the following issues in mind:

- Prepare for what is about to happen, so that *consent and confidentiality* are clearly addressed.
- Prepare what will happen if *something unforeseen* comes up, for instance strong emotions and unplanned topics.
- Prepare for time to *debrief*.
- Debrief carefully after the interview. How did it feel for the one who was interviewed? Did any new thoughts or feelings come up about the interview? Make sure you set aside some time to discuss.
- How did it feel to be the interviewer? What reactions arose for you? Log your own thoughts, feelings and bodily reactions.

Once you have completed your interview, it needs to be transcribed. On the first reading of the transcripts, begin by attempting to 'list every expression relevant to the experience' (Moustakas 1994: 120). Is there a 'moment of the experience that is a necessary and sufficient constituent for understanding it'? If so, 'is it possible to abstract and label it?'

Space does not allow us to enter into the stages of analysis very deeply with regard to any of the methods. Those of you who would like to develop a more in-depth knowledge about phenomenological investigation are advised to approach it through some of the more accessible guides – there are many to choose from.

Finlay and Ballinger (2006: 23) conclude that 'there are myriad possible theoretical perspectives ... social constructionism, structuralism, feminism, critical theory, phenomenology ... the list goes on. These are not just isolated theories. They determine the course of the research and the quality of style of the findings. They also link back to particular methodologies and philosophy.'

Case study

Finlay and Ballinger (2006: 24) offer an example of how a phenomenological and a social constructionist approach will highlight different aspects.

- From a *phenomenological* perspective, the focus on Kenny, 'a male research participant who withdraws to his bedroom', moves to an understanding of subjective experience and consciousness:

  Locking himself in his bedroom, [Kenny] hides from a suddenly threatening world. ... The change in his 'being-in-the world' [...] – his altered consciousness and existence – is confusing and frightening. Past aims and projects have been derailed while the future becomes profoundly uncertain and bleak. (Finlay and Ballinger 2006: 24)

- In the case of 'illness', a *social constructionist* framework on 'Kenny' adopts an understanding of his actions which can be reflected upon in terms of the social, cultural context in which he lives:

  Kenny's performance can ... be understood as a way of 'doing' masculinity [...]. His struggle to respect himself through finding a work role needs to be seen in the context of the stigma arising in his working class community from being an unemployed man who is not fulfilling his family breadwinner role. (Finlay and Ballinger 2006: 25)

Peering into the mind

Emotions are certainly a nebulous subject to study. We have looked at claims for certainty in Freud's work as well as evidence-based theory regarding emotions and the mind. We have viewed options in what could qualify as 'more feebly lit areas', with the hope of finding what we might be missing through a focus on our perception, thinking and feeling about reality, rather than on reality as such.

Frith (2007: 16) muses over the 'the inevitable interaction' which he often dreads at parties. In an anecdote from a social gathering with scientists,

Frith (2007) refers to a suspicious silence which can follow when we tell someone about our profession. The 'Aha, you're a therapist' often followed by the '...and what do you actually do?' Frith (2007: 16) continues:

> This time the question comes from a cocky young man with no tie, probably a nuclear geneticist. 'You're a psychologist? So can you read my mind? ... Wouldn't you rather do real science?

The sly remark reflects a 'hierarchy' within science. So-called hard evidence and science involves aspects which can be measured. Frith continues (2007: 3–4):

> 'Hard' relates to the subject matter of the science and the sort of measurements that can be made. ... You don't believe that speed of light is 299,792,458 metres per second? Here's the equipment. Measure it yourself.' Once we have used the equipment to make the measurement, the numbers come from dials and print-outs and computer screens that anyone can read .... The top sciences are 'hard' while those at the bottom are 'soft'. Confronted with [the] precision of measurements, I have to admit that psychology is very soft.

The evidence-based approach positions psychological treatments closer to the 'hard science' camp than before. The optimism regarding measurement and certainties in the field of psychological treatments reflects, argues Frith (2007: 3–4), a desire to measure.

The emphasis on measuring has been fuelled by the merger between cognitive psychology and neuroscience since the 1970s. The Nobel prize-winner Eric Kandel (2006: 8) concludes that we actually, finally, *can* peer into the human brain:

> Cognitive neuroscience has ... developed ways of 'peering inside the human brain and watching the activity in various regions as people engage in higher mental functions – perceiving a visual image, thinking about a spatial route, initiating a voluntary action.

Instruments like Positron-emission topography (PET) and functional magnetic resonance imaging (fMRI) make it possible to measure the brain's consumption of energy and its use of oxygen. The merger between psychology and molecular biology allows scientists to examine how we think, feel, learn and remember on a molecular level. Kandel (2006: 8) celebrates 'the new science of mind':

> Imbued with new knowledge and confidence, biology turned its attention to its loftiest goal, understanding the biological nature of the human mind. ... The result has been a new science of mind, a science that used the power of molecular biology to examine the great remaining mysteries of life. ... [E]ach mental function in the brain – from the simplest reflex to the most creative act in language, music, and art – is carried out by specialist neural circuits in different regions of the brain.

But is peering inside the human brain the same as reading minds? Frith brings us back to the underlying issue about what it means to be a human. Can we capture the essence of the mind and consciousness in terms of neurons? The humanists at the party (in Frith's case, a professor in English) argue that we can't. The issue about what makes human beings feel, think, judge, reflect – the 'cogito', as Descartes called it – has been debated for as long as we can tell. This ontological stance, i.e. our word view and understanding of the basis for our being, is still a matter for dispute and causes Frith (2007: 15) to celebrate the progress in psychological science with caution:

> So, the problem with psychology is solved. We no longer need to worry about soft, subjective accounts of mental life. We can make hard, objective measurement of brain activity instead. ... [B]ack at the party I can't restrain myself from telling them all about the big science of brain imaging. The physicist quite likes this new development. But the Professor of English doesn't accept that studying brain activity can tell you anything about the human mind ... I move off to refill my glass. I don't argue.

A culture war

The evidence-based approaches may constitute the basis for official guidelines for psychological therapies today, but underneath the surface have been conflicts of opinion – at times to an extent which Messer (2004: 580–81) calls a 'culture war':

> For the past decade there has been a culture war raging over the value and even ethical imperative of ... evidence-based practice ... I use the term culture war because the controversy taps into broad worldviews in matters psychological that divide many [practitioners]. These outlooks include ... subjectivism versus objectivism ... hermeneutics versus universalism ... ideographic versus nomothetic ... and qualitative versus quantitative methods.

Subjectivism, hermeneutics, idiographic and qualitative methods are, writes Messer, anchored in 'humanistic outlooks'. The issue of world view and what we hope to generate knowledge about is captured at Frith's party scenario. The humanist becomes an inevitable party pooper at events where universal truths are being claimed. Bite-sized explanations, i.e. reductions of complex issues such as thoughts, feelings and reflections, can be argued to be so complex that the bite-sized certainties or 'accumulated fragmentalism' (Kelly, in Chiari and Nuzzo 2010: 3) on offer become misrepresentative, in some cases even meaningless.

Rather than arguing about right or wrong, it is probably more constructive to emphasise the importance of being as clear as possible about one's point of departure and framing of the problem.

Evidence and different grounds for belief

The actual meaning of the word 'evidence' is 'ground for belief or disbelief' (McLeod 1987). While we tend to think of evidence as facts or reliable truths, the term 'evidence-based' ultimately refers to communicating clearly the grounds on which we infer and hold something as true or false. Solms and Turnbull (2002: 55) stress 'how important it is for scientists to be aware of the philosophical positions they have adopted'. Philosophy, continue Solms and Turnbull (2002: 55), reminds us, for instance, about how 'it is appropriate to describe certain neuronal processes as causing consciousness only within a particular philosophical framework'. The question regarding, for instance, whether the mind is a muscle or something more can be answered differently depending on our starting point. Frith's example from the party , the 'Professor in English', approaches reality with a different focus from the neuroscientist Kandel, who adopts a realist stance inspired by 'materialist-monism' guided by the belief that our mind ultimately is reducible to physical matters. Solms and Turnbull (2002: 56) adopt an almost Kantian-approach when they argue that we can 'never literally perceive the stuff we are made of without first representing it through one of our perceptual modalities.' Assuming that we are only able to make inferences from the data of our perceptions, continue Solm and Turnbull (2002: 55), our picture of the mental apparatus with inferences of how it works will always be a 'figurative one – a model'. Solms and Turnbull (2002: 55) conclude:

> This graphically illustrates how important it is for scientists to be aware of the philosophical positions they have adopted.

Postmodern critique

Alvesson (2002: 3) asserts that 'there is no independent reality out there, which can be perceived and measured'. Any form of understanding, or 'any gaze' takes place 'through the lenses of language, gender, social class, race, and ethnicity'. Alvesson (2002: 4) continues:

> The great faith in data and empirical inquiry ... has been challenged by a multitude of intellectual streams. ... A powerful one is what may be referred to as 'non-objective' interpretivist perspectives [that claim] that there is no clear window into the inner life of an individual. Any gaze is always filtered through the lenses of language, gender, social class, race, and ethnicity. ...

Alvesson (2002: 4) asserts that 'social science is notoriously political' and that it is no longer possible to approach research about people and society shielded by an objective and neutral approach:

The fact that human interests and cultural, gendered and political ideals put their imprint on methodological ideal, as well as on research practices and results, makes it very difficult to see science as a pure activity, neutral and objective in relationship ... to institutions and interests. Nowadays, it appears in many camps as old-fashioned, intolerant and theoretically and philosophically unsophisticated to favour this kind of idea in parts of social science...

Feminist critique has been particularly influential. Feminist theory addresses male domination of masculine standards, and has now become a methodology in its own right (Dawson 2009). Feminist theory is also a branch within Critical Theory, which explores power issues and 'interest-laden aspects' of social enquiry, and highlights how 'human interests and cultural, gendered and political ideals put their imprint on methodological ideal', as Alvesson (2002: 4) puts it:

[C]ritiques have been raised by feminists pointing to how male domination of masculine standards [such as objectivity, neutrality, distance, control, rationality and abstraction] influence dominant epistemology and methodo-logy in social science. ... [C]ritical theorists emphasize the political and interest- and value-laden nature of social enquiry. ... Even more profound are the views from discursive and constructivists denying science and any privileged access to the objective truth about the social world outside lan-guage and language use. ... Language constructs rather than mirrors phe-nomena, making representation and thus empirical work a basically problematic enterprise.

The umbrella of approaches summed up as 'postmodern theory' has devel-oped in response to the growing critique against universal truth and a priori realities. Alexandrov (2009: 32) refers to 'the anxious awareness of the fallibility of our knowledge [that] marks our time'. This captures the underpinning belief in postmodern theory.

Epistemological straitjacket

In his research about gay couples, Aguinaldo (2004) refers to an 'epistemo-logical straitjacket' of the traditional positivistic outlook. Gay movements, feminism and cross-cultural approaches stress how philosophy presumes a heterosexual male, 'white middle-class individual as the ideal standard' (Parker, cited in Costa 2012: 141). As suggested with reference to Isha's research into black issues in counselling training, mixed-methods and plura-listic approaches are increasingly called for when entering into hitherto neglected and unchartered areas. In an earlier chapter, Beverley Costa shared her experiences of mixed methods in the context of multicultural therapy. In the case study below, this research is put into the context of Beverley's own background and experiences.

Case study

Beverley Costa (2012: 138) established a therapy service to provide a multi-ethnic counselling service which she found was missing. Beverley grew up in a dual heritage family 'surrounded by cultures, which were very different from the mainstream external environment in which we lived'. The impact of migration and the loss of a homeland, the 'acculturation stress', was something which Beverley felt was particularly inappropriately met through traditional therapeutic models and services. Beverly (Costa 2012: 138) continues:

> There were a number of complexities and tensions which faced my family, including acculturation stress, the impact of migration and the loss of a homeland for political reasons, and tensions between the cultures within the home and outside the home.

Beverly found that although black and minority ethnic (BME) communities were overrepresented nationally in services for mental health care via the police or Accident and Emergency services, they were 'starkly underrepresented' in therapeutic forms of care. Beverley (Costa 2012: 138–41) continues:

> In fact statistically, although black and minority ethnic (BME) communities are overrepresented nationally in secondary services for mental health care, their routes of access are normally via the police or Accident and Emergency services as a result of a crisis. They are starkly underrepresented in primary mental health service. ... In all of my training as a psychotherapist, I was left with a sense of dissatisfaction that the models of therapy presented failed to take into account people's different worldviews and migration experiences. The models of therapy on offer in mainstream services tended to be based on an individual-centred worldview and ignore the experience of people from collective-centred cultures. ... At first glance, the philosophy that underpins, for example, the person-centred approach may seem universal. However as Ian Parker (2007: 114) reminds us: 'All models of the mind in psychology are culturally specific', which presume the white 'middle-class individual as the ideal standard'. ... To provide a culturally sensitive, linguistically appropriate and relevant counselling service to members of the black and minority ethnic (BME) population we need to respond to their specific social and psychological needs in a manner which takes into account their expectations and values.

Beverley's work and research highlights how 'the mind in psychology is culturally specific [and presumes] the white 'middle-class individual as the ideal standard'. Her research departs in the social constructionist framework, which emphasises the impact of socio-cultural aspects on what we call self and the mind.

Reflection

How does the idea of a 'white middle-class individual as the ideal standard' relate to your experience of therapy training? If possible, discuss in pairs.

Can you think of other 'voices' which are left unheard, or perhaps misrepresented through what Aguinaldo (2004) refers to as the 'epistemological straitjacket' of traditional ways of making sense of 'reality'?

Fishman (1999) represents one of those researchers who converted from an objective to a non-objective interpretive perspective. 'I first fell in love with the natural science vision in 1958 when I majored in psychology as an undergraduate at Princeton', explains Fishman (1999: 5):

> This [natural scientific] vision fit perfectly with the times, since the 1950s were in many ways the height of the worldview of 'modernism'. Modernist thinking, and the 'positivist' philosophy that underlies it, places a particularly high value on reason. ... Natural science is viewed as a specifically privileged, objective, 'value-free' means for uncovering the true, underlying nature of the physical and human world, independent of our minds and culture.

Fishman (1999: xxii) writes about his frustration over bite-sized certainties, or what he refers to as 'thousands of laboratory-like studies being generated by the field [with] frustratingly little impact upon major social and psychological problems'. Fishman, too, regards the interpretive outlook on knowledge as something which grew in response to a social and political diversity:

> [T]he stability, optimism, self-discipline, and conformity of the 1950s was broken by the 'counterculture' revolution and political upheaval of the 1960s. The changes in the '60s were associated with the emergence of an interrelated family of alternative visions called by such names as 'postmoderninsm', 'neopragmatism', 'social constructionism', 'deconstructionism', 'cultural criticism', 'hermeneutics', and 'antifoundationalism'. ... In spite of popular nostalgia for the 1950s, contemporary media has also exposed their dark side. After all, racism, homophobia, sexism, poverty ... social injustice and environmental pollution ... were hidden from view.

Postmodernism is almost by definition a slippery concept. Rosen and Kuehlwein (1996: 38) wisely conclude that:

> Anyone who thinks he or she knows exactly what postmodernism is and can offer a clear, precise, and coherent definition to demonstrate this knowledge is probably mistaken. ... I mean this not as criticism but as a characteristic. Postmodern theories are self-consciously and self-reflexively aware of this.

They continue, however, with a unifying theme within postmodern thinking:

> Perhaps the one unifying theme ... is that there does not exist an immutable truth in the 'real' world to serve as a bedrock or grounding upon which knowledge can be built. (Rosen and Kuehlwein 1996: 38)

Fishman (1999: 5) approaches postmodernism with reference to framings and lenses, akin to our emphasis earlier on reflective practice and reflexivity:

> [Postmodernism implies that] it is never possible to take the glasses off altogether and view the world as it 'really is', with pure objectivity. All we can do is change glasses and realize that different pairs provide different pictures and perspectives on the world.

Some of the most unifying themes within postmodern research are 'foundationlessness' and 'fragmentariness'. Foundationlessness rests, as Fishman (1999: 5) puts it, on the notion that:

> that there is no objectively knowable external reality that forms a foundation for knowledge, but rather that all knowledge is partial and limited to one of many possible perspectives, consisting of constructions based on human organizing capacities.

Fragmentariness reflects, in turn, the idea that the real is not a single, integrated system, but rather a collection of disunited, disparate elements and events (Fishman 1999: 5).

Constructivism and social constructionism

Constructivism involves, as Fishman (1999: 51) says, 'the notion that human knowledge is not a mirrored reflection of reality, but rather a constructed interpretation "of the experience"'. Rosen and Kuehlwein (1996) conclude that there are many strands within constructivism. The overarching belief within constructivism is, however, that people are 'meaning making creatures and they will spin their web of meaning throughout, all of the time'. This stand moves us closer to idealism than realism. Rosen and Kuehlwein (1996: 5) continue:

> [T]here are a variety of constructivist models, they all hold in common the epistemological belief that a totally objective reality, one that stands apart from the knowing subject, can never fully be known. ... They reject the postulate that our mental representations mirror an objective reality, 'out there' ... rather, knowledge, and the meaning we imbue it with, is a construction of the human mind ... meaning and reality are created and not discovered.

Social constructionism takes the constructivist perception of reality one step further. Constructionism highlights how there are 'common materials, building blocks from which identities and relationships are constructed' (Miell and Dallos 1996: 101). As Miell and Dallos put it:

Rather than seeing people as inevitably free to construe the world in their personal and subjective ways, social constructionism proposes that in any given culture there are common materials, building blocks from which identities and relationships are constructed. (Miell and Dallos 1996: 101)

The outer world is, in this context, not only a mere construction, it is a reality. As Miell and Dallos (1996: 101) highlight:

It is not simply suggested that there is a 'real', objective world 'out there', but that there are dominant beliefs, explanations, ways of thinking about the world, and in particular a shared language which constructs how we see the world. The fact that these socially constructed views continually change does not mean that at any given moment or point of history they do not have a real existence as influential shared ideas.

The case study below illustrates another study which is conducted within the framework of social constructionism. Aguinaldo (2004), who opposes today's 'epistemological straitjacket', practises within health psychology. He explores the impact of ideological and political structures on the way we perceive 'health' within gay male relationships. Aguinaldo (2004: 132) refers to his study in terms of 'qualitative research through a social constructionist lens'. With parallels to Beverley and Isha, Aguinaldo addresses the narrow white, heterosexual Western male-dominated framework. Aguinaldo (2004: 131) explains that to say one is 'promoting health, leaves unexamined potentially problematic functions of "health"'.

Case study

Aguinaldo's (2004: 132–4) study explores 'the conditions within which these gay men entered into their abusive relationship, their experiences and identification of abuse, and the eventual termination of their relationship and subsequent living and surviving after abuse'. He found that 'their accounts were riddled with experiences of pain and suffering inflicted not only from their abusive partners but also from a heterosexist society that refused to acknowledge their victimisation'. Aguinaldo (2004: 132) continues:

Although it is clear that victims of same-sex partner abuse must narrate their experiences consistent with battered wives in order to make their abuse recognizable to others …, such efforts potentially conceal the needs of victimized gay men who do not neatly fit into heterosexualized relationship norms. … An overwhelming majority of the participants initially did not name their experiences of relationship violence as abuse because they did not know 'what abuse is' or 'what it looked like'. It is for this reason that I produced 'case studies' … of their experiences. … The research findings thus functioned as a realist narrative that other gay men

(Continued)

(Continued)

could use to evaluate and assess their own experiences of relationship violence; and to an extent, the narratives produced had accomplished that goal. ... Although the interviewees believed themselves speaking from a universal position of 'a victimized gay man', it was clear to me that their narratives reflected the experiences from a particular social location ... their narratives of abuse spoke little about culturally inappropriate social services that many gay men of colour or new immigrants may have faced.

Viewed from the social constructionist lens, Aguinaldo (2004: 132) considers the narratives of his research participants in the context of how 'medical sociologists have long argued that "health" cannot be invoked as an impartial truth claim':

For example, medical science had once pathologized black slaves for attempting to escape their white masters .... In this sense, 'healthy' black men were once conceived as those who remained subordinated by white supremacist rule. Political resistance to that rule (e.g., black slaves fleeing white supremacy) was viewed as a form of sickness – drapetomania. 'Health', like 'truth' – and thus, validity – can be used as a means to maintain unequal social relations; and consequently, the social conditions that render black men 'unhealthy'. To say one is 'promoting health' as a foundation for the assessment of validity leaves unexamined potentially problematic functions of 'health'. For this reason we need to assess and interrogate validity with an explicit focus on how it operates discursively within social science research. ... By drawing attention to these political structures, the narratives I created functioned as a critical account, however, with only a narrow glimpse of one of a host of social structures that shaped the participants' experiences.

Activity

Aguinaldo argues that one of the functions for research is to address injustice, inconsistency and unequal distribution of power. Do you agree?

Recommended reading

Greco, J. and Sosa, E. (1999) *The Blackwell Guide to Epistemology* (Blackwell Philosophy Guides). Oxford: Blackwell.

This book offers a good insight into epistemology, both its traditional meaning and later developments.

TEN What is reflexivity?

Practice-based research is never conducted in a vacuum. Underlying personal and cultural expectations, values and beliefs (held by both the researcher and the research participants) are inevitable aspects of research conducted in real-life settings. In this chapter, we consider reflexivity as a way of incorporating implicit and explicit, conscious and unconscious aspects of the research process without losing sight of scientific 'rigour'. Particular attention is paid to what Finlay and Gough (2003) refer to as the 'five variants' of reflexivity.

- Emotional agility
- Reflexive awareness
- Dialectical engagement with an 'other'
- Defamiliarisation
- Critical realism
- Feminist research
- Emancipatory research approach
- Unconscious processes
- Methodological 'horrors'
- Subjectivity
- Introspection
- Intersubjectivity
- Mutual collaboration
- Social critique

There are no set ways of defining reflexivity, yet it is increasingly becoming an inevitable aspect of practice-based research. Fox et al. (2007: 157–8) refer to reflexivity as something which helps us to 'habitually' consider the researcher's own impact on the research:

> Reflexivity means that at every stage ... the practitioner has influenced, consciously or unconsciously, the process and has been influenced in turn by the research process. ... Practitioner researcher should habitually stand back from their activities and examine reflexivity at every stage of decision-making in relation to the operation of the research.

Fox et al. (2007: 158) offer an example of practice-based reflexive reasoning with reference to the NHS-based practitioner 'Joan'. She conducts an inquiry into 'how attitudes of the healthcare professionals impacted upon the behaviour and experience of the service users with a history of self-harm'. For Joan, some of the stages of the reflexive process will be to consider the following questions:

- How will her personal interest and experience of self-harm have impacted her interest in researching the subject?
- How has she selected what to read, and how has her reading been shaped by her unique experiences and understanding of practical work with this service group?
- How has her reading informed her thinking about her practice?
- How have decisions about the form of research been influenced by other people's research in the field?
- How can her experience of service users inform her choice of method for the study?
- Who might be rendered vulnerable in the study, and why?
- On what basis has she connected with 'voices' and 'stories' of individuals in the context of what Fox et al. (2007: 156) describe as 'historic, structural and economic relations in which they are situated'?
- What challenges might very different audiences pose to the presented analysis? How will she engage with these challenging viewpoints? Who might she be afraid will see her analysis, and why?
- And so on.

Like postmodern and the non-objective, interpretive approaches in general, reflexivity is often traced to feminist research. Feminist research highlights, as Alvesson (2002: 3) says, how 'male domination has produced a masculine social science built around ideals such as objectivity, neutrality, distance, control, rationality and abstraction [and offers] alternative ideals, such as commitment, empathy, closeness, cooperation, intuition and specificity'.

There is a sensitivity and openness which is typical for reflexivity; a degree of emotional agility is required in ways which moves us more into the 'touching and feeling' stages of searching that we referred to earlier. Etherington (2004: 19) asserts that reflexivity builds on skills which are part of the repertoire of a counsellor:

> Reflexivity is a skill that we develop as counsellors: an ability to notice our responses to the world around us, other people and events, and to use that knowledge to inform our actions, communications and understanding. To be reflexive we need to be aware of personal responses and to be able to make choices about how to use them. We also need to be aware of the personal, social and cultural contexts in which we live and work and to understand how these impact the ways we interpret our world.

Etherington (2004: 19–20) suggests that reflexivity is a relief – almost like 'coming out':

> Over the past 15 years or so, with the challenge created by feminist and new paradigm research methodologies, the use of 'self' has become more and more legitimate in research. [R]eflexivity has become central to my work. ... This has been almost like a process of 'coming out' for me. ... Using reflexivity in my own research has meant I have had to find ways of being openly creative, and this has stimulated me to generate new ideas to help me avoid the research data being poured into a given theoretical mould.

Etheringon (2004: 31) concludes that 'reflexivities' is a more appropriate term, given that there are different approaches to reflexivity:

> For some researchers, reflexive awareness may involve little more than a means of checking against possible sources of subjective bias creeping into an experiment or survey. ... For others, reflexivity may become the primary methodological vehicle for their inquiry.

Bolton defines reflective practice as a stance to learning characterised by reflexive awareness. Bolton (Bolton, cited in Gardner 2006: 145, my italics) writes:

> [Reflective practice] is an approach in which the learner is encouraged to be as *reflexively aware* as possible of their *social*, *political* and *psychological position*, and to question it, as well as their environment.

Dialectical engagement with 'the other'

However, Qualley (1997) stresses that reflexivity takes reflection one step further. She contends that while reflection 'assumes that individuals can access the content of their own mind independently of others', reflexivity relies on a dialectical or critical engagement with an 'other' – and that it is this aspect which makes reflexivity so powerful. Qualley (1997: 11) writes:

> Reflexivity is a response triggered by a dialectical engagement with the other – an other idea, theory, person, culture, text, or even another part of one's self, e.g. a past life.

It is the openness to 'alteration' that provides reflexivity with such power or impact; it usually leads to some form of transformative learning. Qualley (1997: 61) continues:

> [D]uring the dialectical process of trying to comprehend or understand an other, one's own beliefs and assumptions are disclosed, and may themselves become the object of interpretation, critique, and even metamorphosis. It is this risk of

alteration to one's view of the world that makes this kind of [research] dangerous, but also valuable. If the [researcher] is not at risk, his or her current understanding and self-awareness remain safely immune to further complication and illumination.

As suggested earlier in this book, reflexivity invites us to try on new perspectives long enough to gain new angles on familiar frameworks. Carter and Gradin (2001: 5–4) explain: 'By dialectical we mean the back-and-forth interplay of opposing ideas. ... Reflexivity, then, involves trying on the perspective, the world view of an "other" for long enough to look back critically at ourselves, our ideas, our assumptions, our values.'

Activity

Stuart and Whitmore (2008: 156) refer to reflexivity in terms of its broad interest in how the 'knower's presence ... influences what is known and how this occurs'. Consider a research scenario where you are interviewing ten businesswomen about their 'risk taking' in business. Six women are white, middle-class women and one of these women is heavily pregnant. Another woman speaks with a strong Mancunican (Manchester) accent, one woman is Afro-Caribbean, another comes from Sweden and one woman wears a burqa.

- Choose one aspect of your own 'subjectivity' (for instance, your gender, ethnicity, social background, sexual orientation, physical ability, age, ethical framework, emotions, cognitive and theoretical constructions) and consider at least two ways in which your subjectivity might impact on the way the women approach the subject of 'risk taking' and the way you might 'hear' them.

Defamiliarization

As suggested earlier, reflexivity involves a 'dialectical engagement' with 'an other', as Qualley (1997) puts it, 'for long enough to look back critically at ourselves, our ideas, our assumptions, our values'. Defamiliarization is an example of attempts to address the distinction between interpretation and reality; it is a strategy aimed at challenging the 'habitualization of perception' which usually follows our routine interaction with people and experience.

Activity

Return to the interview scenario, but approach the prospect of interviewing the businesswomen with different 'subjectivity' criteria from your own gender, nationality, social background, etc. If you are young, female or working-class, consider what it could be like to approach the interviews as a much older person, or as a man, or maybe from another social or cultural background.

Reflexivity represents 'an effort to reflect upon how the researcher is located in a particular social, political, cultural and linguistic context' (Alvesson 2002: 179), and to work on the assumption that there are many 'truths'. The validity of our research rests on being as transparent as possible about the way we have gone about selecting, collecting and analysing, etc. The researcher becomes, as Finlay and Gough (2003: 5) put it, 'a central figure who actively constructs the collection, selection and interpretation of data':

> [W]e appreciate that research is co-constituted – a joint product of participants, researcher and their relationship. We realise that meanings are negotiated within particular social contexts so that another researcher will unfold a different story. (Finlay and Gough 2003: 5)

Critical realism

A not unusual epistemological positioning within practice-based research with a reflexive stance is the 'critical realist' perspective. Critical realism reflects the belief that, as Etherington (2004: 71) puts it, 'the world exists there independently of our being conscious of its existence [but that] it becomes a world of meaning only when meaning-making beings make sense of it'. This view positions the reflexive researcher in between realism and idealism, as we addressed earlier.

The term 'critical' is, as suggested earlier, used in research that challenges the 'taken for granted' within social contexts. Critical researchers are, as Finlay and Ballinger (2006: 258) assert, 'concerned with unpacking how concepts come to be constructed as common sense, and exploring the social implications of such common and unproblematic views'. Finlay and Ballinger (2006: 20, 258) write:

> Critical realism ... acknowledges there is a pre-existing reality and that it is the purpose of social enquiry to explore this. It also recognises that this reality is mediated through and by individual experience and representation, and is socially situated. [...] Critical realist researchers tend to be pragmatic. They consider meanings to be fluid ... accepting that participants' stories of having an illness do reflect something of their subjective perception (if not their actual experience).

Most critical research involves some form of 'deconstruction' and involves finding loopholes and inconsistencies in the realist explanation. In this sense, critical realism involves some form of 'unpacking' of results, with an interest in political, cultural or psychological aspects of our meaning-making processes. There is a critical, subversive and emancipatory approach; it questions what we hold as 'real'. Feminist research and multicultural research are examples of research which takes oppressive and power-related issues into account. Others choose to focus on psychological aspects, as in the case of Hollway and Jefferson (2000), who research with an interest in unconscious processes.

Doing practise-based research informed by reflexivity

'Situatedness' (Costley et al. 2010: 1) is, as suggested, the hallmark of practice-based research:

> Situatedness arises from the interplay between agent (you, the researcher), situation (the particular set of circumstance and your position within it) and context (where, when and background). Organizational, professional and personal context will affect the way a piece of research is undertaken.

We looked earlier at how real-life research challenges the traditional understanding of 'methodological horrors' (Parker et al. 1994: 10). As Parker et al. (1994) assert, it should be possible to follow a piece of research, repeat it even, but not with exactly the same outcome as the basis for its validity. An intrinsic part of the research process is 'how the subjectivity of the researcher has structured the way [the exploration] is defined in the first place', assert Parker et al. (1994: 13). They continue:

> Subjectivity is a resource, not a problem. ... When researchers, whether quantitative or qualitative, believe that they are being most objective by keeping a distance between themselves and their objects of study, they are actually themselves producing a subjective account, for a position of distance is still a position and it is all more powerful if it refuses to acknowledge itself to be such.

It has been argued in this book that the emotional aspects of the relationship between researcher and their research participants play a significant part in what we call 'knowledge' in practice-based research in the field of therapy. Yet, this kind of knowledge tends to be generated 'in feebly lit areas and by touching and feeling'.

How to do it?

In this section, reflexivity will be explored in more depth. Finlay and Gough (2003: 5) write:

> [W]e now accept that the researcher is a central figure who actively constructs the collection, selection and interpretation of the data. We appreciate that meanings are co-negotiated within particular social contexts so that another researcher will unfold another story. ... In short, researchers no longer question the need for reflexivity: the question is 'how to do it?'

This section is a response to the question about 'how to do it?' The debate about reflexivity 'inhabits', as Finlay and Gough (2003: 5) put it, claims made by researchers of different theoretical persuasions with regard to the rational and practice. As suggested earlier, Finlay and Gough's (2003: 6) 'five variants of reflexivity' offer a helpful overview. Pursuing the focus on the emotions in research, we have decided to concentrate on the first three forms of reflexivity, namely introspection, intersubjectivity and mutual collaboration. The distinction is fleeting and reflects a different emphasis and focus, while all three share the overarching aim of using the researcher's own experiences to inform the research process and outcome. Reflexivity is neither about purging nor self-awareness as such. Reflexivity is, as Etherington (2004) points out, legitimised on the basis that it is believed to contribute something to the study. Where emotions are playing a part of the research, reflexivity helps us to conceptualise 'how our own thoughts, feelings, environment and social and personal history inform us as we dialogue with participants, transcribe their conversations with us and write our representations of our work' (Etherington 2004: 32).

Five 'variants' of reflexivity

Finlay and Gough (2003: 6) identify five 'variants' of reflexivity, with regard to shifting aim and focus on introspection, intersubjectivity, mutual collaboration, social critique and ironic deconstruction. These approaches will be reflected in the research examples later on in this book. We will particularly return to reflexivity on introspection, intersubjectivity and mutual collaboration. Social critique and postmodern deconstruction are, however, of underlying importance, given the guiding belief in this book about there being 'local' truths rather than one universal truth about reality.

- **Reflexivity on introspection**: This reflexive stance involves an emphasis on the 'value of self-dialogue and discovery' to 'embrace the humanness as the basis for psychological understanding [or use] introspection to yield insights which then form the basis of a more generalised understanding and interpretation' (Finlay and Gough 2003: 6–7).
- **Reflexivity as intersubjective reflection**: The researchers 'explore the mutual meanings involved in the research relationship' (Finlay and Gough 2003: 6); the self-in-relation to others becomes 'both focus and object of focus'.
- **Reflexivity as mutual collaboration**: Researchers use reflexivity to 'hear, and take into account, multiple voices and conflicting positions' in order to 'move beyond their preconceived theories and subjective understanding' (Finlay and Gough 2003: 11).
- **Reflexivity as social critique**: Of particular importance here is how to manage the power imbalance between researcher and participant. Researchers adopting this stance will 'openly acknowledge tensions arising from different social positions, for instance, in relation to class, gender and race' (Finlay and Gough 2003: 12).

- **Reflexivity as ironic deconstruction**: This reflexive stance is usually linked to the social critique. It has developed from researchers adhering to the post-structuralist and postmodern critique of modernism and its claim for universal truth. The ironic method of deconstruction 'lays bare a hidden but decisive weakness in the text under study'. As Alvesson and Skoldberg (2000: 154) put it, 'we turn things upside down, and make the hitherto oppressed side the dominating one'. In this form of reflexivity 'attention is paid to the ambiguity of meanings in language used and to how this impacts on modes of presentation' (Finlay and Gough 2003: 12). Rather than assuming that language mirrors the 'reality out there', researchers adopt the stance that language conveys social and historical distinctions which 'provide unity and differences' (Alvesson 2002: 53). Language tells us that there are workers, managers, employed and unemployed; each category comes with a set of values and beliefs, which researchers may challenge by more careful use of language, for instance by an ongoing attempt to 'defamiliarize' themselves and 'avoid seeing the social world as self-evident and familiar' (Alvesson 2002: 91).

Recommended reading

Denzin, N. and Lincoln, Y. (2005) *The SAGE Handbook of Qualitative Research.* London: Sage.

This book is a classic for beginners with an interest in how research methodology 'works' and has developed over time.

ELEVEN   Reflexivity on introspection

This chapter builds on research where reflexivity on introspection is being adopted, for instance, with reference to real-life examples of heuristic and autoethnographic research.

- Introspection
- Immersion
- Self-examination
- Heuristics
- Ethnography
- Creative writing
- Journaling

This chapter revolves around self-reflection and self-awareness in research. The category which Finlay and Gough (2003) refer to as 'reflexivity on introspection' is illustrated in Figure 11.1. Reflexivity on introspection assumes that paying attention to the researcher's own reactions will add to the research. Almost like the strip of Litmus paper that changes colour in chemical experiments, our researcher will react and respond to her environment, and these reactions can be logged and reflected upon. This stance assumes that there is a 'personal connection with the topic of inquiry, which inevitably leads to self-examination, significant personal learning and change' (Etherington 2004:110), and these changes are incorporated into the study.

Heuristic research is referred to by Finlay as an example of introspective reflection. Whereas phenomenology, as Moustakas (1990: 38) puts it, 'encourages a kind of detachment to the phenomenon being investigated, heuristics emphasize connectedness and relationships'. He refers to person-centred theory and to Carl Rogers' emphasis on the self and one's 'internal frame of reference' to conceptualise meanings of an experience, and as part of the 'dialogue between oneself and one's research participants' (Moustakas 1990: 39). To recreate the lived experience 'fully and completely', different

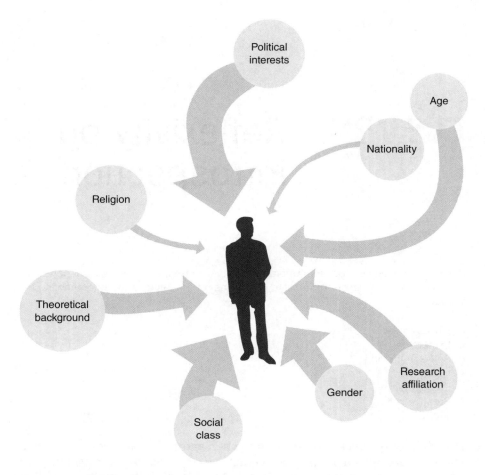

Figure 11.1   Introspection (drawing by Finbar Charleson)

means of expression play an important role, including poems, artwork, diaries, autobiographical logs and other personal documents. The research process starts, however, with a firm focus on the researcher to 'yield insights which then form the basis of a more generalised understanding and interpretation' (Finlay and Gough 2003: 6).

Barber (2006: 3) writes that 'as the researcher is the most important inquiry tool in Gestalt-informed research, then "you" becomes a subject worthy of research'. Barber (2006: 3) emphasises the 'need for you to describe the mental-set and the position you are starting out from':

> I feel I cannot stress too strongly the need for you to describe the mental-set and the position you are starting out from, for changes of this will provide evidence of how the research field is impacting you.

Claire Asherson Bartram has researched mothers in stepfamily situations. Her research resulted in a dissertation entitled 'Narratives of Mothers in Stepfamily Situations: an Explorative Investigation' (Asherson Bartram 2009). Claire's research journey illustrates how heuristic inquiry can be applied in practice-based research. In extracts from her dissertation, Claire (Asherson Bartram 2009: 49–64) reflects over how she regards research and psychotherapeutic practice as overlapping interests (see case study below).

Case study

I can remember as a child wanting to be understood by my parents. I thought 'if they know how I feel then they would understand'. This now transfers to the stance I hold as a therapist and researcher: 'if I know how they feel then I will understand'. However, neither is entirely true; I can never fully know another person. What I can know is how I respond to another person as my inner world is influenced by what is outside me.

As a researcher, I have clues towards recognising or understanding another person's experience through my own senses, i.e. sight, hearing, touch, emotional feeling and reactions. I recognise what is 'out there' through what I directly experience 'in here' inside of my own skin. While I cannot be inside another person, there are times when my reactions in their presence give clues to what they are going through. For example, I might feel sad and heavy when I am with somebody who is grieving, or excited and enlivened as I hear someone talking with enthusiasm. Such responses can bring about a powerful sense of connection; a moment when I and another person recognise each other as feeling, experiencing beings. The moment which Martin Buber describes as a movement from an 'I–it' relating to an 'I–thou' meeting, where I–it represents separation and 'I–thou' represents connection (Buber 1958).

Barber (2006: 3) emphasises the importance of keeping a research journal where both ideas and feelings are recorded. In heuristic inquiry 'autobiographical and "meditative" come especially to the fore', writes Barber (2006: 78), and the researcher is encouraged to 'travel ever deeper into his/her inner experiences of a theme'. Moustakas' (1990, cited in Hiles 2001) 'stages' of the heuristic inquiry (see Figure 11.2) captures the different levels of reflection.

Moustakas refers, for instance, to the starting point in terms of a 'passionate concern that calls out to the researcher' and regards the research process as something which 'is lived in waking, sleeping and even dream states'. Stages of 'incubation', 'illumination' and 'explication' involves a 'preparatory phase of solitude and meditation' which leads the researcher

> **Initial engagement**
> The task of the first phase is to discover an intense interest, a passionate concern that calls out to the researcher, one that holds important social meanings and personal, compelling implications. The research question that emerges lingers with the researcher, awaiting the disciplined commitment that will reveal its underlying meanings.

> **Immersion**
> The research question is lived in waking, sleeping and even dream states. This requires alertness, concentration and self-searching. Virtually anything connected with the question becomes raw material for immersion.

> **Incubation**
> This involves a retreat from the intense, concentrated focus, allowing the expansion of knowledge to take place at a more subtle level, enabling the inner tacit dimension and intuition to clarify and extend understanding.

> **Illumination**
> This involves a breakthrough, a process of awakening that occurs naturally when the researcher is open and receptive to tacit knowledge and intuition. It involves opening a door to new awareness, a modification of an old understanding, a synthesis of fragmented knowledge, or new discovery.

> **Explication**
> This involves a full examination of what has been awakened in consciousness. What is required is organization and a comprehensive depiction of the core themes.

> **Creative synthesis**
> Thoroughly familiar with the data, and following a preparatory phase of solitude and meditation, the researcher puts the components and core themes usually into the form of creative synthesis expressed as a narrative account, a report, a thesis, a poem, story, drawing, painting, etc.

> **Validation of the heuristic inquiry**
> The question of validity is one of meaning. Does the synthesis present comprehensively, vividly, and accurately the meanings and essences of the experience? Returning again and again to the data to check whether they embrace the necessary and sufficient meanings. Finally, feedback is obtained through participant validation, and receiving responses from others.

Figure 11.2 The stages in an heuristic inquiry: an example of reflexivity on introspection (Moustakas 1990, in Hiles 2001: 3–4)

onto a 'creative synthesis', continues Moustakas (1990, cited in Hiles 2001: 3), where the researcher 'puts the components and core themes usually into the form of creative synthesis expressed as a narrative account, a report, a thesis, a poem, story, drawing, painting, etc.'. A significant aspect of the heuristic inquiry is the 'validation' phase; a final stage, which involves feedback from the research participants regarding the interpretation. 'Does the synthesis present comprehensively, vividly, and accurately the meanings and essences of the experience?' asks Hiles (2001: 4). The inquiry usually involves a level of collaborative inquiry, where the interviewee is invited to react to and offer their input to the final interpretive work.

Claire (Asherson Bartram 2009: 49–64) refers to the 'heuristic process' as what 'framed the implementation of this project'. In the following extracts, Claire illustrates how she has used 'Heuristic Inquiry (Barber, 2006), alongside a description of research activities, edited journal entries and other writing, to show how I have experienced being a "research tool".'

Case study

Extracts from 'Narratives of Mothers in Stepfamily Situations: An Exploratory Investigation (Asherson Bartram 2009: 49–64)

... This section is intended to illuminate some of what the research has personally entailed; the heuristic process which framed the implementation of this project. I recorded this aspect of my work in a journal which was a mixture of free writing about how I was feeling, or ideas and themes, dreams that connected how I was experiencing myself within the research, snippets of overheard conversation and notes taken during seminars and meetings.

I have used Moustakas' description of the six stages of Heuristic Inquiry (Barber, 2006), alongside a description of research activities, edited journal entries and other writing, to show how I have experienced being a 'research tool'.

Stage 1 – Initial Engagement

Paul Barber:

The researcher immerses his/herself in a deep personal questioning of what precisely he/she wishes to research, in order to discover and awaken an intense interest, relationship and passion in the research subject (p. 78).

Activities:

- setting up a pilot cooperative inquiry group on stepfamilies
- writing the first draft of my learning agreement, which is not accepted
- abandoning this first course of action
- identifying the research question
- re-writing my learning agreement, which is accepted.

Journal entries:

Why Stepfamilies? Why this Subject at this time? The quick answer is that my family is a stepfamily and that seems important to me. ...

I gather together a group of therapists and lay people to explore stepfamilies.

... On reading my notes, I notice that my anxieties seem to relate entirely to stepfamily issues. My concerns are about how people who were in the first

(Continued)

(Continued)

group will get on with people who are in the second one. I have written: 'I am no longer focused on stepfamilies, I am more concerned about the group and how the new people will fit in.' Reading this now, I recognise how this echoes the concerns a mother might feel, introducing new stepfamily members to her children.

On being given the feedback that a focus on Stepfamily Dynamics is too broad, I have decided to focus on part of the whole picture by interviewing mothers like myself. ... By choosing this focus I have put myself right in the middle of this investigation. It thereby becomes a self-investigation that extends from me to the wider world. It will answer a core query of whether I am alone in finding mothering in a stepfamily situation painful. ...

Comment:

At this stage I am beginning to do explorative activities connected with my future project.

... It took me a while to decide on the focus of mothers – an area less all-encompassing than 'stepfamily dynamics'. In so doing, I have brought the entire project closer to issues that touch my heart.

Stage 2 – Immersion

Paul Barber:

The researcher begins to live, sleep, dream and merge with the research question to the extent that he/she becomes it, so as to appreciate its intimate effects from the inside (p. 78).

Activities:

- I am interviewed by Debbie
- I interview other women, listening intently to their stories and becoming more involved in thinking about what they are telling me
- I transcribe several interviews and then delegate this work to other transcribers
- I listen to recordings of the interviews and correct the transcripts
- I edit the transcripts to make first-person transcripts – very absorbing work
- I run a workshop for the British Gestalt Society.

Journal entries:

I am dreaming about my ex-husband. [etc.]

Claire's research illustrates, again, how reflexive research involves listening to, and linking, what is outside with what is inside the person who is doing the research. Claire addressed several important questions, for instance how her role in stepfamilies seems to link into her role in other groups:

> On reading my notes I notice that my anxieties seem to relate to ... how people who were in the first group will get on with people who are in the second one. I have written: 'I am no longer focused on stepfamilies, I am more concerned about the group and how the new people will fit in'. ... [T]his echoes the concerns a mother might feel, introducing new stepfamily members to her children.

Claire also describes how her research focus develops in response to feedback from outside and how this choice helps her to address 'a core query of whether I am alone in finding mothering in a stepfamily situation painful'.

Her notes illustrate also the researcher's struggle with finding an appropriate methodology. Claire muses: 'Is it acceptable to present a patchwork doctorate with a mixture of methodologies? ... Can I justify this?'

Journaling

Journaling is a consistent and significant aspect of this kind of research, not only in terms of personal awareness, but as a way to meet the requirement of 'specificity' (Parker et al. 1994). As explored earlier, real-life research does not claim its validity on the basis of 'replicability', as research conducted within the framework of traditional natural sciences does. The validity of the research is rather linked to whether the research process can be traced, repeated even – albeit with the different character that each unique researcher clearly brings to the research. Costley et al. (2010: 33) conclude:

> It is ... important to your own perspectives or premises clearly, that is to state your personal model of understanding of a situation. The process of articulating your own position will allow others to reflect on other constructions. Subjectivity, in this sense, is unavoidable...

This 'process of articulating your own position' gives transparency and accountability a slightly different meaning compared with evidence-based research. It invites the outsider to follow the researcher's journey and decide for themselves where they consider different actions could be taken; and personal development becomes an inevitable part of this.

Journaling plays a significant role in reflexivity on introspection, and since it captures so much of the personal development, many choose to include parts of it in the final research thesis.

Typical for reflective journaling is the 'feedback loop' in the writing; it involves returning to our writing with a reflective response in mind rather than 'purging' or telling it 'as it happened'. The reflective journal involves transformative learning experiences. Contrary to popular belief, few people write a comprehensive text at their first attempt, so don't feel despondent if your journal entries fail to make much sense. Smith (1991) suggests that any readable text requires three stages:

- Prewriting: scribbling or note taking.
- Writing: this can be in the form of uninterrupted writing or writing that starts with a prompt, an idea, a feeling or an association.
- Rewriting: this involves an 'editorial' return to the text, with a particular reader group, theme, plot, structure or general interest in mind.

One way of rewriting with the feedback loop in mind is to return to the text after the prewriting or the writing and offer feedback concerning the content and the feelings that the text have evoked. There are, as Thompson (2011: 35) describes, 'two types of feedback statements':

1. Feedback about your content, like

   ○ When I read this I notice ...
   ○ When I read this I get surprised by ...
   ○ When I read this I remember ...
   ○ When I read this I realize that ...

2. Feedback about feelings, like

   ○ When I read this I get a sensation of ...
   ○ When I read this I feel ...
   ○ When I read this I am aware of ...

Relative permanence

Writing can help us both to access and consider events and experiences more easily than in everyday speech. Writing brings an element of *'relative permanence'* (Smith 1991) to our meaning-making processes; it 'freezes' (Bolton 2005) moments of our thinking and helps us view our thought processes as if on a film. We can linger with and return to the way we understand and organise events and experiences.

Comments about writing

Ironically, a not uncommon sensation after first attempts at reflective writing is a sense of failure, frustration or emptiness. There is often a general miscomprehension about the writing we produce, as if it ought to convey something worth reflecting upon right from the start. This can be as hard as co-ordinating two different movements at once, particularly if we have a strong inner 'critic' who expects our writing to be 'good' from the first draft. Dorothea Brande suggests that we think in terms of 'the two persons of the writer' (1934/1996: 44):

- The *unconscious* must flow freely and richly, bringing at demand all the treasures of memory, incidents, scenes, intimations of character and relationships which it has stored away in its depths. The unconscious will provide the writer with 'types' of all kinds, typical scenes, typical emotional responses ...

- The *conscious* mind will 'edit', i.e. control, combine, and discriminate between the materials 'without hampering the unconscious flow'.

Cameron (1998: 11) has coined the phrase 'writing for the hell of it can be heaven'. She refers to stages when 'the writing writes through the writer' rather than the other way around:

> When we forget ourselves, we when let go of being good and settle into just being a writer, we begin to have the experience of writing through us. When we are just the vehicle, the storyteller and not the point of the story, we often write very well – we certainly write more easily.

Activity

Put everything else to one side for the moment and write for five minutes about whatever comes into your head. Below are three alternative prompts to choose from, if you need that to get started:

- Focus on something 'small' in your immediate surroundings. Dust on a lamp shade or a shadow in the corner of the room, etc., *or*
- Focus on a feeling – perhaps cold feet, a wound on your finger or maybe a noise from outside. For instance, 'There's a dog barking outside, he sounds hungry/lonely/cold/excited ...', *or*
- Write for five minutes with the following opening: 'He reached out his hand, and when it almost touched ...'

Relaxing the watch to the gate of Reason

Freud wrote about the importance of 'relaxing the watch by the gate of Reason' (Freud 1900/1976: 177). He compared free, uninterrupted writing with dreaming and emphasised the value of free association and to allow our thoughts to arrive 'pell-mell' (Freud 1900/1976: 177). The first draft can be the most exciting and exhilarating to write; it can be like opening a tap and can lead us to places and encounters that we least expect. However, the first draft can also be a disappointment to read. I often feel as if only half the story is caught on paper in my first drafts. Still, if we accept that our stories will need revisiting to become reader-friendly, creative writing lends itself as an excellent route into our inner world. According to Bolton (2005: 5):

> If we had asked people to talk about their values in abstract terms, we would have received responses. By asking them to tell [write] stories about important experiences, we were able to see something of how values reveal themselves in a complex, varied and shifting way in practice.

Autoethnography

Autoethnographic research involves using the researcher's own experiences as a route into the understanding of others. Ellis and Bochner (2000, cited in Trahar 2009: 7) define autoethnography as a 'genre of writing and research that displays multiple layers of consciousness, connecting the personal to the cultural'. They continue:

> Back and forth autoethnographers gaze, first through an ethnographic wide-angle lens, focusing outward on social and cultural aspects of the personal experience; then they look inward, exposing a vulnerable self that is moved by and may move through, refract and resist cultural interpretations.

Etherington (2004: 126) concludes that the heuristic approach has 'been criticized for its inward focus that does not address the more outgoing dialogue and culturally embedded relationship between researcher and the researched'. Autoethnography puts the introspective in a cultural context. Ethnography has, as Ethertington (2004: 140) writes, 'traditionally focused on the "other" as an object of study, typically spending time observing people in other cultures and societies'. Chang (2008) brings a reflexive focus into the research and encourages a focus on how the researcher's own cultural biases might impact the research.

An example of an ethnographic study, where the researchers 'use their own experience as a route through which to produce academic knowledge', is Pink's research about sensory experiences (Pink 2009: 64). For instance, how does smell impact the way we understand the reality we live in? Pink approaches realist assumptions about our five senses from several angles. Pink uses the term 'sensory subjectivity' and 'sensory biases'. She explores, for instance, the experience of housework with reference to smell, and to what people find clean or not. Pink (2009: 51) asserts that:

> An important step towards understanding other people's sensory categories and the way they use these to describe their experience, knowledge and practice lies in developing a reflexive appreciation of one's own sensorium.

She builds on her 'own subjective decisions about laundry' to access the understanding of 'how the way one treats laundry is bound up with how one creates statements about self on the basis of sensory categories':

> I have been doing laundry myself for many years, yet found that my knowledge and embodied ways of knowing about laundry, and ways of interpreting the domestic environment in relation to laundry processes differed – sometimes enormously – from those of the people who participated in my research.

By comparing her own experience with the experience of others of, for instance, 'clean', Pink find that smell, touch, seeing, etc. means different things to different people. Pink (2009: 52) continues:

Their (varied) beliefs and values concerning how one should use one's senses to judge when and in what ways laundry was clean or dirty led me to a different consciousness about how I made my own subjective decisions about laundry. However, this self-reflexivity also allowed me to understand how the way one treats laundry is bound up with how one uses sensory categories and practice to create statements about one's self-identity.

Pink (2009: 53) identifies differences between people with regard to their ideas of what 'clean' is in terms of 'identity markers ... such as gender, sexuality, ethnicity, age and generation' (Pink 2009: 53). These identity markers develop in the context of culturally imposed models and values linked to vision, smell, etc. With this in mind, Pink (2009: 52) advocates a greater 'sensitivity to a multiplicity of sensory expressions' and challenges our own Western categorization of five senses. Researchers have tradition-ally adopted a realist assumption about smell, touch, hearing, sight and taste. Sensory ethnography contends that sensory expressions are invested with cultural values and meanings:

> In much research methods literature produced originally in the English language, the 'we' who do research are assumed to be modern western subjects, who divide the sense into vision, hearing, touch and smell (along with the often added mysterious sixth sense). Howes and Classes, stress that 'other cultures do not necessarily divide the sensorium as we do'. ... [T]he Hansa have two senses and the Javanese five. ... The Western model of five senses is a folk model ... and, as such, it is one among others. (Pink 2009: 51)

Generating knowledge for the research becomes, in this way, a process which involves an 'emplaced, sensorial, and empathetic' involvement rather than neutral observation. The autoethnographic researcher hopes that 'the similarities and continuities between her or his own experience and those of others can lead to an understanding of how it feels to be emplaced in particular ways' (Pink 2009: 63). This idea is illustrated in the research by Edvardsson and Street (2007, cited in Pink 2009: 67) about 'how different environments affect ways of provision and an understanding of care'. By increasing the sensory and embodied nature of their own experiences, they hoped to access different types of sensory experience of others:

> While being at the ward as a participating observer, DE found that he instinc-tively joined in the brisk pace habitually used by the nurse as they moved around at the unit. ... He found that the brisk movement and sound of the hurried steps of staff prompted the sensation of wanting to move with the pace of the unit. ... [This] led him to understand the way that corridors were used in these units as spaces for passage and not for lingering or chance encounters. ... This epiphany stimulated his curiosity to explore further how people moved around the unit and what this movement might mean. (Edvardsson and Street 2007, cited in Pink 2009: 67)

Activity

The case study below illustrates Guy Harrison's research on 'Spiritual and Pastoral Care within the NHS Health Trust'. He is considering using his own experience as a chaplain/therapist 'as a route through which to produce academic knowledge', as Pink (2009: 64) puts it. Guy explains his research concerns, and argues for some of the strengths and weaknesses in autoethnography as a suitable approach for his research.

- Can you think of any examples where autoethnography and the idea of using your own experiences as a route into the situation of others might benefit your own research?

Case study

An introduction to autoethnography (Guy Harrison)

The focus of my research is an evaluation of my practice as Head of Spiritual and Pastoral Care within an NHS Health Trust. Within this role I seek to combine my training and experience in person-centred therapy with my training and experience in pastoral care. It is a personal story researched through an in-depth, single, narrative case study of practice, set within an autoethnographical frame.

Autoethnography is an approach to research and writing that seeks to describe and systematically analyse (graphy) personal experience (auto) in order to understand cultural experience (ethno). By adopting this approach the aim is to produce research that is grounded in personal experience and alerts readers to the cultural and values-laden institutional context in which the researcher exercises their role.

Autoethnography combines characteristics of both ethnography and autobiography. Autobiographers write about remembered moments that have impacted on their lives and which they wish to bring to the attention of others. Such experiences are usually selective and retrospective and may include journal accounts, photographs and video recordings as well as interviews with significant others. Autobiographers will often recollect images, feelings and memories which may derive from either experiences of existential angst or revelatory insight.

Typically, ethnographers are social scientists who study the practices, values and beliefs that are held in common and which are shared within a particular cultural context. They do this by becoming participant observers, by taking field notes of what is happening and the relationships that exist within a given context. Ethnographers are concerned to develop a comprehensive description and understanding of a given context and as such are concerned about all aspects of the way people live their lives.

Autoethnography in research about therapy

In a counselling and psychotherapy context McLeod suggests that as a research approach, ethnography 'is uniquely capable of capturing the quality and characteristics of the "lived interactions" between therapists and client' (McLeod 2001: 68). Bringing the 'self' into ethnography and making it autoethnography is a developing field within counselling and psychotherapy research. It particularly appeals to therapists who are trained in humanistic approaches and who use congruence and/or self-disclosure as a way of assisting clients to tell their particular story.

How autoethnography fits into my research

My aims in adopting an autoethnographic approach are to:

- provide an authoritative practitioner voice within the chaplain/therapist role
- make a particular contribution to this role
- enable understanding of the hierarchical and professional boundaries that influence the scope and purpose of the role
- provide a unique health care chaplaincy perspective on the role
- provide an alternative source of ideas for the development of theory and further research.

My rationale for choosing this methodological approach reflects the fact that whilst numerous studies of pastoral care exist and the relationship with counselling and psychotherapy is often referred to, they bear little resemblance to the role I inhabit. None of the published research captures the experience of caring for patients and how contextual influences shape and constrain such care. ... This lack of integration provides the impetus to research my own experience.

Critique and response

One criticism of the authoethnographic approach is to suggest that by focusing on myself in this way I run the risk of shaping the production of the data in such a fashion that I could be said to be producing what I expect to find.

In order to address this risk, the approach has reflexivity as a central component. Reflexivity is a way of making transparent my values and beliefs as they affect my interpretations and as they consequently influence the research process and its outcomes. By engaging reflexively, Etherington (2004) suggests that researchers ensure rigor and improve the quality and validity of research. By adopting a reflexive approach to my experience and therefore my writing, by using different narrative styles, such as poetic form, by seeking to tell my story and analyse that story, I am attempting to affirm not only my identity as a chaplain/therapist but also actively engage and challenge others to do the same.

Guy brings the question of faith and therapy to the forefront. He wants to critically explore the prospects of combining a training and experience in person-centred therapy with the training and experience of pastoral care. It is, he concludes, an unchartered territory. His own experiences can contribute to what Pink (2009: 53) refers to as 'identity markers' and means of understanding 'how an individual is positioned in relation to social institutions and other individuals'. A distinct interest in autoethnography is, as Pink (2009: 53) addresses, how 'we continuously move and learn, with the effect that our self-identities are continuously reconstituted'. It is in this sense not just a matter of identifying one's values, beliefs and biases at the start of the research, but perhaps primarily about using experiences as points of reference on an ongoing basis, i.e. as something which grows and changes during the process. Pink (2009) and Edvardsson and Street (2007) illustrate this aim, as they record the development of their own values throughout the interaction with their research participants.

Autoethnography aims in this sense to use the researchers' responses as a point of reference to cultural differences and a route into cultural situatedness of different experiences.

Recommended reading

Muncey, T. (2010) *Creating Autoethnography*. London: Sage.

This is an accessible and insightful guide to the different stages of autoethnographic research and writing.

TWELVE Reflexivity as intersubjective reflection

This chapter examines intersubjective processes in research. It emphasises psycho-analytically informed research, where transference, countertransference and 'unconscious' processes are part of the process.

- Psychoanalysis
- Transference
- Countertransference
- Unconscious processes
- Psycho-social research
- Emotions
- Ongoing consent
- Infant-observation model
- Free-association interview

Introspective and intersubjective, and indeed collaborative and politically informed, reflexivity are interlinked and related. Typically, what Finlay and Gough (2003: 6) refer to as a form of reflexivity based 'on intersubjective reflection' is that researchers 'explore the mutual meanings involved in the research relationship'. As highlighted in Figure 12.1, the self-in-relation to others becomes 'both focus and object of focus' (Finlay and Gough 2003: 6).

This is not dissimilar from the autoethnographic approach, which bridges introspective and intersubjective reflexivity. We will return to the issue of ethnography below, although with an emphasis on transference, countertransference and unconscious processes.

Psychosocial research can, as Clarke and Hodgett's (2009: 2) explain, 'be seen as a cluster of methodologies [which] considers the unconscious communications, dynamics and defences that exist in the research environment'.

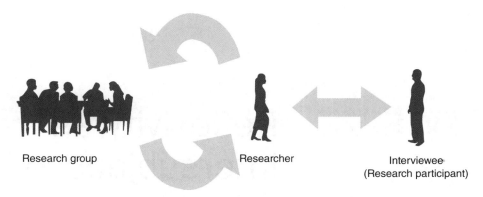

Research group   Researcher   Interviewee
(Research participant)

Figure 12.1 Intersubjectivity (drawing by Finbar Charleson)

Psychosocial research is based on 'the notion that the unconscious plays a role in the construction of our reality', and that this 'plays a significant part in the generation of research data and the construction of the research activity' (Clarke and Hodgett 2009: 2).

The psychosocial research brings projection, transference and counter-transference to the forefront. Hollway and Jefferson (2000: 93) refer to an 'unconscious intersubjective dynamic' where 'we are influenced by our emotional responses'. Hollway and Jefferson (2000: 45) continue:

> This means that both will be subject to projections and introjections of ideas and feelings coming from the other person. It also means that the impressions that we have about each other are derived simply from the 'real' relationship, but that what we say and do in the interaction will be mediated by internal fantasies which derive from our histories of significant relationships. Such histories are often accessible only through our feelings and not through our conscious awareness.

Hollway and Jefferson (2000: 43) are often referred to in the context of the psychosocial approach. Their theory on the 'subject' suggests that we incorporate anxiety and defensive functions in our research:

> Psychosocial research adopts a theoretical starting point [to] construe both researcher and researched as anxious defended subjects, whose mental boundaries are porous where unconscious material is concerned.

Using emotions to inform the research

Projections in the research relationship can, argues the psychosocial researcher, work both as a resource (through, for instance, identification, recognition and containment), and an obstacle; they can trigger defences and misunderstandings in the interview. The following extract illustrates how an unconscious intersubjectivity enters the research relationship in terms of mother–daughter dynamics. Hollway and Jefferson (2000: 48) write:

> Jane and I were both white ... our class difference was stark ... I was probably close to the age of Jane's mother. I think it was this structural feature of our identity which precipitated the unconscious dynamics of which I got a glimpse in my unease about leaving Jane at the end of the second interview, [and when] Jane trailed off, I felt responsible for keeping the interview going.

As in Claire's heuristic research earlier, Hollway and Jefferson are recognising and bringing their own emotional response into the research. Also, with parallels to Guy's autoethnographic research, there is an aim to understand the research participants through one's own reactions.

Activity

'Consent', 'choice' and 'decision' are ambiguous terms in this kind of research. Hollway and Jefferson (2000: 88) refer to 'doorsteps decisions', which are likely to be informed by first impressions and fantasies rather than a rational, considered decision. 'The decision to consent, then, cannot be reduced to a conscious, cognitive process but is a continuing emotional awareness', write Hollway and Jefferson (2000: 88). They therefore agree with Josselson (2011) (see Chapter 7 on ethics). Consent becomes a subject for ongoing negotiation, and should always involve the option of withdrawing or opting out. Hollway and Jefferson (2000: 89) suggest gaining consent before and after any interaction:

> Typically, the guidelines construe the issue of consent as 'before' and 'after' the research intervention. 'After', for them, involves 'debriefing' to deal with ethical issues which arise from discrepancies between prior information and fuller information which, by implication, it is the right of participants to know at the end.

- How would you, as a research participant, feel if the interview opened up topics which you felt unprepared for? In what way could this level of openness be agreed upon, beforehand, do you think? Are there perhaps limits to consider beforehand, as an interviewer? If so, how would you phrase these?

We looked earlier at Anne Atkinson's research about therapy and abortion. This was based on the 'free association narrative interview' (FANI), inspired by Hollway and Jefferson (2000). Anne used the psychoanalytically inspired interview model in order to provide as much space as possible for the research participant's own associations to develop around a theme.

However, as illustrated by Anne in her research reflections, a free associa-tion is difficult in research (and as her research suggested in response to these experiences, possibly difficult to achieve in therapy too). The researcher's responses will invariably impact the participant, and vice versa, and the method is still under development.

The infant-observation model in different settings

The psychoanalytically informed infant-observation model (Clarke and Hodgett 2009; Hollway 2011; Hollway and Jefferson 2012; Urwin and Sternberg 2012) is becoming increasingly recognised within research as having an intersubjective emphasis. We looked at this approach briefly in the context of Pamela Stewart's research of infants and their mothers in prison. Urwin and Sternberg (2012: 6) explain the basics of infant observa-tion as follows:

> Infant observation ... refers to a method of following a baby's development over time. ... [It was] developed initially by Esther Bick as part of the formal curriculum of the Tavistock Child Psychotherapy course in 1948. ... In the typical situation, an observation student on a course ... finds parents about to have a new baby who are willing to allow an observer to visit them at home regularly, normally weekly [usually] over two years. ... [T]he students tries to take an unobtrusive, non-interfering position, concentrating on the infant and taking in as much as possible of what is happening. ... No notes are taken at the time.

As in the free association interviews, the psychoanalytic infant-observation method puts emotions to the forefront, and suggests that 'emotions, qua emotions, have to be felt in some way, even in a very mild identificatory way, to be faithfully recorded by an observer' (Price and Cooper 2012: 57). An essential aspect of the observation model is, however, its collabo-rative approach to the data analysis. The observers meet regularly to dis-cuss their narratives in 'seminar groups'. Urwin and Sternberg (2012: 6) continue:

> Students are encouraged to make their actual observations as free from theo-retical preconception as possible, and the description of what they have seen often has a spontaneity, even rawness, that may reflect the impact of the obser-vation experience. These narrative accounts are discussed subsequently in a small seminar group ... that meets weekly. ... Over time, patterns in each infant's way of behaving and responding may become apparent. Theoretical ideas may be introduced gradually.

The infant-observation model is, as Shuttleworth (2012: 171) says, 'an ethno-graphic research method' which is being applied in new areas, for instance in the Health sector and in nursing homes:

> In recent years, infant observation has come to be seen not only as part of clinical training, but as an ethnographic research method that gives access to the psychological development of the infant within ordinary family life. ... It has also been used as a research method in new areas of study ... as a wider social research project.

Again, not dissimilar to the autoethnographic research, the psychoanalytical model for infant observation has been adopted in different contexts with the aim of using the researcher's experience as a route into the experience of others.

Below is an extract (Heussler, in Datler et al. 2012: 167) from an observation in a nursing home for the elderly:

> Mrs Gabler now leans in her wheelchair and once again gazes at me. She appears to be content. She burps slightly, and gives a little sigh. 'I don't need much more ... but the coffee was good!' ... She briefly looks away from me, and then back to me. 'But what can I tell you! It's the same thing every day. Always the same ... First I sit here, then they bring in the breakfast', ... Mrs Gabler sighs, 'Well what am I to do. When I was still able to walk, things were different.' There is a pause, and Mrs Gabler appears to be lost in her own thoughts. She then reaches into her pocket of her nightgown and takes out a cloth napkin, wiping her mouth with it. ... Now she gazes at me directly ... and says: 'I've tried everything already, anyway. Not eating anything, not drinking anything. But it got me nowhere. It's going to take a long time with me. My constitution is too good!' I find myself horrified when I hear her say this, and feel a deep sense of empathy and sadness spreading right through me.

In the nursing home for the elderly, the researcher muses over the observed behaviour in the staff and what it feels like to discuss their own very strong emotions while in the nursing homes. By recognising their own defensive processes, their discussion opens up to the emotional response the caregivers may experience – and to the extent to which the organisation allows these to be attended to.

As suggested, the psychoanalytic supervision plays an important part in the infant-observation model, both on an individual level and on a group basis. This supervision is, as Price and Cooper (2012: 64, 60) write:

> less a matter of supervisory 'expertise' and more the provision of 'thinking minds' relatively unaffected by the very phenomena in which we are interested – unconscious dimensions of the field inquiry. [Sometimes] to re-connect the elements of the account and make them coherent or thinkable once more.

Next is another example of how the observation model is being applied in another nursing home by an observer who follows some of the patients whose health is deteriorating for no obvious reason. The emotional responses of the researcher are incorporated as part of the 'data gathering'.

Case study

The observer visits the home weekly and repeatedly records episodes from Mr Hartz's daily life in the home. The following extract illustrates some of Mr Hartz's relationships and the relationships which surround him. Datler et al. (2012: 160ff) write:

'Mr Hartz is a tall, slender, 75-year-old man who suffers from dementia and, for that reason, now lives in a nursing home. During the day he enjoys going for walks through the corridors of the dementia unit, but is otherwise barely able to eat or drink without assistance. His ability to communicate with others is steadily diminishing. ... Mr Hartz is visited by his wife. The observer, Ms Ursula Bog, who visits on a weekly basis, repeatedly records episodes of tender contact between them. ... The 12th observation, for example, illustrates such tenderness.'

Observation notes 1:

'Mr Hartz carefully reaches out towards his wife's hand. He lifts her left hand slightly upward and places it on the table. Mrs Hartz is still talking to the lady, while her husband turns her hand to and fro, again and again. She then slowly reaches for his and holds it gently in hers. Both of them also put their other hands on the surface of the table and stroke each other's hand... etc.'

Observation notes 2:

'Mr Hartz approaches me. He comes up very close in front of me, staring down my cleavage. As he does so, he smiles. He remains standing like this for some time without moving at all, looking at me. The short distance between us eventually makes me uncomfortable, and I take a step back. He comes a step forward, and again stands directly in front of me. Only after Nurse Martha has returned does he retreat from me, and goes to stand by the window.' (Bog, cited in Datler et al. 2012: 164)

There were several observation sessions, but the above illustrate the range of experiences which the observer brought to her seminars. Price and Cooper (2012: 67) reflect:

> In the observers' accounts, there was not a single scene in which nurses or relatives showed any kind of deep interest in Mr Hartz's sexual feelings, desires or fantasies, or of understanding how painful it must have been for him to no longer experience himself as attractive, desirable and potent. After analysing all the reports, the research team concluded that this reflected a common characteristic in the day-to-day experience of all nursing home residents.

The regular research seminars can throw new light and add perspectives to the observer's understanding. The seminars aim also to help the researcher to tease out meanings which remain on an enacted level, yet out of awareness for the observer; particularly when there have been strong emotions involved and the observer might have acted on a 'wish to protect themselves from more intense encounters with the painful emotions'. Price and Cooper (2012: 64) assert that:

> Researchers are exposed to primitive and unprocessed psychic 'material' and will also inevitably identify with research subjects and their ordinary defensive functioning in the field. They will need the help of others who are not so emotionally involved with the material in order to rediscover reflective thinking capacity in relation to unprocessed ... data. This is the function of individual, and especially group, psychoanalytic research supervision.

These experiences are incorporated into the research. Anxiety-provoking and defensive reactions are becoming part of the research 'knowledge'. If the observer might have acted on a 'wish to protect themselves from more intense encounters with the painful emotions', as Price and Cooper (2012: 67) assert, perhaps the research is highlighting something which goes on for the staff as well:

> We were aware that the observers often felt very strong emotions in the nursing homes, or when they discussed the accounts of their observations in the seminars. ... On the other hand, when these accounts were discussed ... it was often difficult for the observers to reflect upon the resident's feelings. ... When this issue was discussed, we came to understand that the observers' behaviour could be an expression of their unconscious wish to protect themselves from more intense encounters with the painful emotions with which the residents of the nursing home often had to struggle. ... This led us as a research team to assume that defensive processes like these were also at work on the part of caregivers. ... In this light, we understand some of the limitations if the quality of the relationships observed between nursing staff and residents are serving to protect staff members from the strength of the barely tolerable primitive emotions constantly aroused when working with demented old people.

To increase 'the containing capability' of the caregiver, the research suggests 'the development of a social space' where the professional 'is permitted – and empowered – to work in a climate in which psychological and social factors are taken into account' (Datler et al. 2012: 169). In other words, the research suggests that the nursing home creates space for the staff to address uncomfortable and confusing experiences. A greater understanding of their own strong reactions, such as disgust, anger, contempt or disinterest, could improve their relationship with the patients. In this sense, the infant-observation model addresses underlying motivations at play in our work. It invites us to address questions around what other people's helplessness stirs in ourselves and how these responses can be used constructively rather than being enacted or displaced. As Hollway (2011: 53) asserts, the infant-observation model aims to 'help turn the emotional experience into thinking':

The psychoanalytic ('infant') observation method includes several layers to help turn the emotional experience into thinking, including the resource of others. The training helps to cultivate the requisite epistemological uncertainty during the observation hours themselves. ...The group's task is to use members' subjective responses to the case, which the group can then reflect upon together. This helps the processing of observers' experiences.

A similar focus underpinned Pamela Stewart's research about mothers and babies in prison. Pamela (Stewart 1998: 3) explains:

The relationship with the mother is central to future development of the infant. This paper explores relationships of mothers and babies in prison and considers how far effective mothering is possible in prison.

Pamela approaches mother–children bonds in prison, with an interest in providing containment for good-enough mothering. As Winnicott (1961) addressed, a good-enough mother needs to be contained in order to provide containment herself. As in previous examples, the infant-observation model is used as a tool to tap into a complex web of emotions. What is it like to be a mother in prison? And what is it like for prison wardens to be with babies and their mothers? What can we learn about the mothers' underlying motivations and about our own reactions to the way the mother–infant dyad is being played out, to provide the appropriate support for mothers to be good-enough for their babies?

Pamela positioned her research within object relations theory. The extracts below capture some of her theoretical understanding with regards to how the mother and infant relationship might impact the child's development.

Of particular significance for Pamela's pre-understanding of infant–mother relationships are the three 'contrasting styles of parental container "shapes"' (Briggs and Behringer 2012: 152), in terms of:

- a 'concave'-shaped containment 'where the parent allows infant communications and states of mind to enter her mind and body'
- a 'flat' containment, often occurring in depressed and preoccupied parents who are 'missing, not noticing or blocking infant communication'
- a 'convex'-shaped containment, where the infant becomes a 'receptacle' for the parent's own preoccupations and states of mind.

Pamela (Stewart 1998: 3–7) explains the way these concepts are being incorporated in her research below.

Case study

The baby, in his primary unintegrated state, needs a mind to hold the parts of his personality together (Bick [1968]). Bick described the mother as providing psychic skin. Through familiar smells, sounds and holding, the baby knits together. If these basic needs are not met, the baby must develop a 'second skin'. Failures in holding results in the baby desperately seeking another object – noise, the television, a light – to pull the parts of his personality together through his own muscular tension. Missing is the mother's mind – the vital magnet to put the fragments of the baby together.

Briggs (1997) continues to explore the concept of containment by formulating three categories to describe the mother–baby interaction. The first, concave shape, is used to describe the mother who is capable of identifying with her baby sufficiently to transform his feelings into thoughts. Concave containment is similar to Bion's concept of reverie.

The second shape described by Briggs is flat. Here the mother ignores the infant's emotions by switching off or focusing on her own experiences. This denies the baby the experience of being thought about and held.

Even worse for development is the convex shape which is reminiscent of the situation described by Segal or Bion's notion of nameless dread. Here the mother adds her own terror and anxiety to the infant's. This is disastrous for the baby who internalises the experience of not being understood – a negation of meaning. A very frequent example in prison is that of the baby being fed. In the convex shape the feeding resonates with force and intrusion, often ending with the baby being sick – forcing the projections back literally onto the mother. In the convex shape the mother's own distress mingles and multiplies, rather than mediates, the baby's distress. The baby experiences this as nameless dread: sensing, but without understanding, that something is wrong. I will use these three categories to think about the mothers and babies I observed, giving the observations as examples or evidence of each type of containment; however, the last two categories (flat and convex) do not seem to be containment at all to me.

Klein observed a baby's keen ability to feel that mother's state of mind impacts on his own mental state. For the baby of an anxious mother, this anxiety compounds his own. This is frequently noted in many observations in more traditional settings. The added anxiety in prison makes a huge impact on the mother and also on the baby.

Even very young babies attempt to deal with the mother's anxiety. One way to avoid these feelings is for the baby to deny them by going flat and appearing cut off. Bion and Klein described the process of extreme projective identification or protection though omnipotent phantasy. Winnicott described the false self. Bick talked about this as a second skin formation. All of these defences cause confusion between real, objective events and subjective experience .... This confusion is a huge impediment to learning how to think.

In the convex situation the infant's experience of the mother is damaging to the development of a reflective, thinking self in touch with reality. The likeliness of this increased with a postnatally or chronically depressed [mother], exhibiting symptoms of 'pervasive low mood, irritability, anxiety poor concentration' ....

Being in prison impacts on a mother's capacity to engage in the development of thought and thinking characteristic of reverie's concave shape. Given that even ordinary, external demands (such as financial or domestic pressures) can impact negatively on the mother's mental capacities at times, the anxiety of imprisonment

(Continued)

(Continued)

presents additional problems. The depression in prison militates against what Bowlby saw as the organic and developing relationship between mother and child sustained by mutual responsiveness. Mutual responsiveness is conspicuous by its absence in my observations, or where it can be glimpsed it cannot be sustained.

One of Pamela's conclusions is that prison *can* act as a containing place. Some examples illustrate how the mother has undergone a positive transformation, and how the mother feels contained enough to allow 'infant communications and states of mind to enter her mind and body', as Briggs and Behringer (2012: 152) put it. The case study below offers an example of a 'flat-shaped' containment (Stewart 1998: 4, Briggs and Behringer 2012: 152), where the preoccupied parent is 'missing, not noticing or blocking infant communication'.

Case study

Observation 2 (Stewart 1998: 16)

Flat containment. Martha and Cinnamon (13 months) and Luther (7 months)

Now 13 months old Cinnamon and her mother Martha had been in prison for 10 months in remand. They had arrived at Heathrow and Martha had been followed. The next day, 17 October, in what Martha described as a terrifying police raid she, her daughter and a suitcase full of heroin were seized by the police. Martha had 5 other children at home in the Caribbean. Apart from infrequent, very expensive phone calls to their various schools, Martha has no idea what is happening at home. The children have been farmed out as no one person has taken charge of them. When she was arrested her oldest child was nearly 14.

Cinnamon and Luther were laughing. Cinnamon dropped the rake and reached for a nearby toy spade. Looking back at Luther she smiled again and then crawled close to her mother, Martha, who was sewing. Martha had her back to the children as she worked the machine. Heavily this large woman rose to check the sewing she had completed. Cinnamon grinned to herself as she approached her mother's strong black legs.

With shrieks of glee Cinnamon pulled herself up to standing while holding on to the chair her mother had just left. Happily she began banging on the plastic seat. Very sharply in her heavy ... accent Martha snarled 'You stop that – naughty'.

Then Martha growled 'If you don't stop that I will smack you for yesterday, today and tomorrow.'

Cinnamon continued beating the spade, looking her mother straight in the eyes. The bright moment of play snapped as Martha raised her huge hand to Cinnamon. With the mighty thud of defeat Cinnamon sank down on to the floor. With a quivering glance at her towering mother, Cinnamon, with a sad sigh, threw away the spade – rejecting it as violently as her mother rejected her.

Paradoxically, here we see a mother persecuted by the favourable signs of her child playing. The mother's mind is so full of her own anxiety that she cannot respond in an encouraging, extending way to her own child. Baby observation usually concerns itself with the impact on the baby by the mother. It is important to remember that this is a two-way relationship. Here the impact of the baby's freedom on the mother is one which evokes envy in the mother and the wish to spoil. The mother seems to have internalised the oppressor and passes this oppression onto her child, effectively blocking all the positive projections from Cinnamon in a flat way.

One of the problems with thinking of observation as a science is the absence of a control mother. How do we know how Martha would respond if she were at home with her other children? We do not know; but I suggest she would not, no matter how great the cultural differences … have responded in this violent, blocking, hand-raising manner. If in the pre-prison past Martha had responded in this negative way, it is unlikely that she would have a child still capable of playing in such an unfavourable environment.

While trying to make allowances for cultural differences it was always very difficult to know where a great deal of Martha's violence sprang from since much of it could be understood as coming from the horrible uncertainty facing them both. However, the West Indian tradition of plaiting the children's hair was very difficult to watch. This is a traditional activity and always looks very painful for the babies.

In another extract, Pamela illustrates the third 'shape' of containment, namely the 'convex', where the infant becomes a 'receptacle' for the parent's own preoccupations and states of mind. Pamela (Stewart 1998: 34) observed several examples of this and concludes that:

Often in prison I had observed a reversal of the maternal, protecting role. Instead of mothers providing a protective shield for their baby, the baby was used to protect the mother.

In a couple of cases, the mothers appeared to relate to their babies in a 'fetished way', continues Pamela (Stewart 1998: 34), and she refers to how Welldon (1991) describes a fetish as being endowed with 'sexual significance entirely unsuited to the normal sexual aim'. Pamela (Stewart 1998: 34) continues:

I had the feeling Joe and Dave were being used in this way. Again I was confused: what was I observing – the past, present or future? In keeping with Welldon's description, I felt the mothers were using their babies in an attempt to deal with their own intense, chronic depression which resulted from a very deprived childhood in which (the mother) was made to feel part of her mother's body, existing only to provide her mother with narcissistic or sexual gratification.

These observations were particularly challenging, concludes Pamela. She describes how (Stewart 1998: 34):

> [These experiences make] thinking difficult and observation painful. The healthy cycle of projection and introjection veered off a course, becoming a vicious circle. How did both babies feel? Did they have to sleep to get through the experience of being treated as a sexual part object? Given their ages I might have expected to see more lively, engaged babies. Instead they both appeared flat, cut off and lifeless.

As a final example of the way that Pamela (Stewart 1998: 28–30) refers to differently 'shaped' containments, the extract below illustrates this 'convex' approach, where the infant fills the mother's empty space.

Case study

Observation 9 (Stewart 1998: 28–30)

Convex containment. Marie and Terri (8 months)

The women were eating their lunch in a windowless room. Many were facing the wall. Marie came in with her daughter Terri. Wearing a soiled t-shirt, worn-out cotton bedroom slippers and torn sweat pants Marie appeared dirty and dishevelled. Equally, Terri's pink shorts and shirt were crusty with old food. Terri was wearing only one slipper that looked too small as her foot appeared red and puffy. Even the buggy looked battered, faded and soiled. Terri had been born while her mother was in prison.

Terri was watching her mother carefully. Sitting well back in her buggy, the 9 month old baby at first appeared relaxed, with one leg dangling down, slipperless. Yet the other leg was pulled up into her body, as if for protection. Her finger nails and toe nails looked well cared for in contrast to her grubby clothes.

Marie said she was going to make Terri's lunch. Terri looked at her mother leave and then at me sitting next to her. She started to make little kicking motions with her dangling leg as if marking time until her mother returned. She smiled at me and started to kick harder. This time she touched my knee, looked up and smiled as if happy to make contact.

Coming back into the room I noticed how short Marie looked in contrast to her huge daughter. Terri looked from me to her mother and then at the purple plastic high bowl. Pulling her eyebrows down she seemed to frown briefly.

Marie put the bowl down and settled Terri into the yellow plastic high chair. Terri did not seem to react to being moved apart from stiffening her arms as if bracing herself against a fall. Terri again frowned at the bowl.

There did not seem to be a drink ready, only the bowl. Without putting on a bib Marie quickly started feeding the baby huge, dripping spoonfuls, saying 'This is Weetabix, this has lots of lovely sugar in it, jus' the way you like it...'.

Obediently, Terri opened her smooth pink mouth. In a way which is hard to describe, her mouth seemed to stay open – as if the food was not being fed to her but funnelled straight down into her stomach. This reminded me of the suf-fragettes being force-fed in prison. The food looked like dirty hay. Hot and lumpy it seemed as if it would very hard to swallow without a drink.

Terri's eyes were wide, glued to her mother's face; she was watching her mother not the spoon coming at her. Her mouth looked like a target, a bullseye. As Marie fed the baby, the mother poured her story into me ...

[From after-comments] ... This feeding did have the quality of force. In with the food went all the undigested grief of Marie's own losses of family, sister and absent mother. Terri was indeed looking at ghosts. The horror for me was the sense of seeing history repeat itself, a broken record stuck in a cracked groove with no hope of remedy or repair. Absence of understanding guarantees endless repetition. It seemed as if these tangled feelings would be passed on with no hope of repair or reversal. I thought about repetition compulsion with its implicit lack of choice or change. Being unable to learn from the past and thus con-demned to repeat it seemed like an additional prison sentence, a prison within a prison of the Russian doll image often used to express containment. Without understanding there could be no working through, without a thinking mother I sensed there could be no possibility of reflection or change.

As mentioned with Gabrielle and Luther, some mothers used their babies inappropriately as sources for their own conflict.

Pamela's infant observation involves the options of using the researcher's cognitive and emotional responses as knowledge about emotionally fraught situations and, through this, contributes in areas which otherwise might remain neglected for defensive reasons. Pamela (Stewart 1998: 11) comments on the willingness among the staff to improve their support, and she writes:

> The sensitivity of the prison staff and the openness to my work was an indication of the staff's desire to think about their jobs and the mothers and babies in their care.

Her final conclusions regarding the impact of her study involves reflections on both a personal and professional level. Pamela (Stewart 1998: 37) writes:

> Taking what can be learned from observing might be a way of helping these mothers. Should babies be in prison at all? Certainly maternal deprivation can occur when a mother is physically but not mentally present. Has the time come to extend the containment model?

> I have tried to apply the observational model as a means of gaining access to 'the dispossessed' women in prison. Observation became a means of containing

the anxiety in a way useful to many mothers, babies and, at times, some of the staff. I wanted to use prison as a laboratory to collect data for 'gaining and testing knowledge'. I believe that I found that Bion's model of container/contained is immensely useful in thinking not only about mothers and babies but also as a means for 'understanding our understanding'.

After the gaining and testing of knowledge, then what? ...With knowledge of the importance of containment and the consequences of its failure, is there a way to act, rather than feel that one is merely acting out and thereby failing to contain one's own anxiety?

In the case of Pamela's research, 'to act' is to provide greater psychological support for both mothers and staff. Of particular importance, argues Pamela (Stewart 1998: 14), is to provide therapeutic support for the mothers to understand their own emotions with regard to their own children, for instance in light of how they have been brought up themselves. Pamela (Stewart 1998: 36) concludes that the prison setting obviously can act as a compound of difficulties:

Prison is a place of pain, emotion, awash with emotion and often violence. Screaming, banging, the throwing of sanitary towels from windows, suicide attempts and self-harm are part of prison life. It is an environment which places the mothers, their babies and the staff at risk.

However, during her two years as an observer, she also recognised different sides of the prison setting. One of the potentials of the prison setting is its capacity to provide the mothers with an opportunity to understand their emotions and how these are being transmitted into the relationship to their babies. Pamela (Stewart 1998: 14, 36) reflects:

Prison is a social institution and as such can act as a container. To add to the complexity of observing in prison there are times when the prison functions creatively, encouraging growth. Observing would have been easier if the prison had been a consistently thought-blocking institution staffed by unfeeling officers. Prison is a complex institution, not a western film with good guys and bad guys. Much as I yearned to know absolutely who was good and who was bad it was not so clear-cut.

There were many monstrous mothers and extremely sensitive staff. Prison was much more intricate than media reports reflect. The view that there is only crime and punishment and no thinking going on within the prison staff is not accurate. Indeed, if this had been the case my proposal would never have stood a chance. Society seems reluctant to think about prison but this is not true of the prison service.

An American journalist writing of the women on death row in Texas noted that the prison gave the women a sense of childhood they had never known. With the set routine, company of other women, sympathetic staff and protection from abusive partners, some women thrive in prison. Many women thrive on the unit, suffering when the release date approaches. ...

[However] for the babies to thrive, both staff and the mothers need much greater support and thought. It is not enough for society to send mothers away – literally out of sight and out of mind. All prisoners exist in a social context with families left bereft by a system that is failing the society it is meant to serve. Much more thought, political action and psychotherapeutic intervention is urgently required if we are to avoid a future of inmates who were themselves born inside. Greater access to pyschotherapy for prisoners might be one way for psychotherapy to answer its early promise of social change.

Interim reflections

We have by now looked at several different approaches, or what Hollway (2011) refers to as 'accents', within reflexivity. Reflexivity 'with a psycho-analytic accent' emphasises the value in 'recognizing our emotional involve-ment in the project, whether conscious or unconscious', as addressed by Clarke and Hodgett (2009: 7). They continue (2009: 7):

> [A]t the heart of the project [of psychosocial research] is the reflexive practi-tioner... [T]he idea of the reflexive practitioner involves a sustained and critical self-reflection on our methods and practice, to recognize our emotional involve-ment in the project, whether conscious or unconscious. ... Why are we interested in our research project: why choose this area and not some other? What is our investment in it and will this affect the way we go about the research? Importantly, how will the above affect our relationship to the subject(s)?

Evaluation and change

When practitioners 'get involved in research', writes Robson (2002: 201), 'they often want to change something in their practice'. This has been the case in the autoethnographic and the infant-observation models in particu-lar; they both illustrate a common form of practice-based and 'real world research' in the form of an 'evaluation'. There are at least 100 types of evaluation, contends Robson (2002: 204), who continues:

> Much real world research in the social sciences has the main purpose of evalu-ating something. Real world researchers also often have ... hopes and inten-tions that the research and its findings will be used in some way to make a difference to the lives and situations of those involved.

Recommended reading

Hinshelwood, R.D. and Skogstadt, W. (2000) *Observing Organisations: Anxiety, Defence and Culture in Health Care*. London and New York: Routledge.

This book offers a psychoanalytically informed understanding of healthcare organisa-tions based on participant observation.

THIRTEEN

Reflexivity as mutual collaboration

This chapter concerns collaborative research. It asks who is being heard, and why? We look at real-life examples of co-operative inquiry into school-based therapy in socially deprived areas and the role of black issues in counselling training. The chapter includes examples of how to invite and run co-operative inquiry groups.

- Action research
- Co-operative inquiry
- Reflexive response
- Inconcludability
- Power
- Pluralistic approach
- Grounded theory

This chapter revolves around research that emphasises the value of a collaborative problem formulation and search process. The researcher raises questions about who is being heard, and why, and incorporates this interest in meaning-making processes throughout the study (Figure 13.1).

In this final chapter about reflexive approaches, evaluation is a particularly pronounced theme. We will look at two different attempts to evaluate a practice: Isha Mckenzie-Mavinga (2005) explores the role of black issues in counselling training through 'pluralistic' research, and Stephen Adams-Langley (2011) describes how he evaluates school-based therapy through 'grounded' theory. Both examples fall within a framework referred to as action research. According to Finlay and Balinger (2006: 257), *action research* addresses 'the specific aim of improving the quality or performance of an organisation or a service'. Typical of this kind of research is that the researcher is participating in the organisational change while doing the research, for instance, Isha incorporates 'black issues' in the training where she already works.

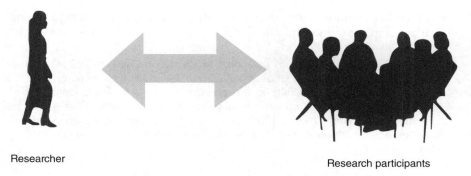

Researcher   Research participants

Figure 13.1   Collaboration (drawing by Finbar Charleson)

Costley et al. (2010) suggest there are two forms of collaboration in practice-based research: collegial collaboration, such as the infant-observation model which is incorporated through regular research seminars; and collaboration between researchers and participants. Sometimes, as we shall see in Isha's case, the two may overlap.

Collaborative inquiry is congruent with the practice-based philosophy that knowledge is co-created. An insider's perspective will inevitably be influenced by his or her environments, and much of this book has revolved around the potential of using this as an advantage rather than, as the traditional positivist approach assumes, as an obstacle. There is, as we saw earlier, always an element of 'inconcludability' (Parker 1994: 13) in real-life research:

> An account can always be supplemented further. There will always be a gap between the meanings that appear in a research setting and the account written in the report, and that gap is the space for a reader to bring their own understanding ... to bear on the text. While a positivist will see inconcludability as a fatal problem, qualitative researchers who follow the change in meanings in the course of research will both understand and welcome the opportunity for others to supplement their account.

Who is being heard, and why?

In this section our focus will move to research where supplemented understanding is particularly welcome. When Finlay and Gough (2003: 164) refer to reflexivity as mutual collaboration, they approach collaborative inquiry in terms of it being 'rooted in social constructionist and post-structuralist epistemologies [focusing on] the ideological nature of knowledge [with an] emphasis on the social world as a site where power relations are played out'.

Meanings are, continue Finlay and Gough (2003: 164), 'always disputable depending on who is speaking to whom and the power relations either held or perceived to be held within these interactions'. In collaborative inquiry, the researcher positions him or herself within a group to answer questions which are important to them all. Yorks and Kasl (2002: 93–5) write:

> Collaborative inquiry resets on principles articulated by Reason (1994) and Heron (1996) when they write about a process that they now call co-operative inquiry. [...] Instrinsic to co-operative inquiry are two fundamental participatory principles. First, each inquirer participates actively in his or her own meaning-making by using processes that ground new knowledge in personal experience. Second, each inquirer participates fully in all decisions that affect the inquiry.

Heron (1996: 14) describes 'knowing' as a 'mutual awakening', and contends that *'knowers can only be knowers when known by other knowers'*.

Knowing develops, continues Heron (1996: 14), in 'participation, through meeting and dialogue, in a culture of shared language, values, norms and beliefs'.

A study of black issues in counsellor training

The collaborative focus on who is being heard and why invites us to address values and norms in critical ways. Our first example is from Isha Mckenzie-Mavinga's (2005) research into 'black issues in postgraduate training'. Isha Mckenzie-Mavinga describes her research interest in terms of 'integrating black issues' into the counsellor training curriculum. We looked at Isha's research earlier in our chapter about ethical considerations.

Isha (Mckenzie-Mavinga 2005: 1) reflects over being an 'insider outsider' throughout her research:

> The researcher's role as black facilitator, tutor, researcher and 'insider outsider' played an important part in both the challenging nature of this study and a model for developing 'safety' and compassion to facilitate the process.

Reflexivity involves, as suggested, pitting one's understanding against other perspectives. There is an ongoing focus on how we as researchers develop our own understanding in light of personal, cultural, linguistic and theoretical perspectives.

In Isha's research, the focus group formulates, collaboratively at first, a tentative title for the research. Isha explains (Mckenzie-Mavinga 2005: 1) the sense of confusion and unease within the group with regard to how black issues were being approached. The discussions within the focus group caused a re-negotiation of the research question. The initial research question changed from: *Can we use history shared through art and creativity to understand black issues in the therapeutic process?* to: **How do trainee counsellors in Britain understand concerns about black issues raised by themselves during their training or about clients during the therapeutic process?**

A significant issue in this kind of research was to find a method which related to black issues. She refers to how traditional frameworks often convey 'Eurocentric inferences' and she develops a pluralistic approach in response to this gap. Isha's description of the process of finding a suitable theory is set out in the following case study.

Case study

Understanding black issues in postgraduate training (Mckenzie-Mavinga 2005)

I found that [traditional] theory did not implicitly apply strategies to black issues work. Therefore their use could confine the method and impose Eurocentric inferences if applied dogmatically. [...] **Drawing on a pluralistic approach**, the heuristic process of understanding trainee counsellors' relationship with the phenomenon of black issues was explored during training workshops. The study gave voice to trainee counsellors' concerns. It encouraged dialogue about relationships as black people, or with black peoples, that link to the therapeutic process. [...] Within this paradigm I drew on elements of Qualitative Multicultural Action research [and] a Heuristic [approach], placing an emphasis on the experiential process and needs of trainees [with a focus on] Narrative inquiry [guided by] the importance of listening to trainees' voices in their natural form. (Mckenzie-Mavinga 2005: 1)

Isha worked with both trainers and students. Isha's primary data 'was created by introducing the phenomenon of black issues into the counselling course curriculum through workshops' in order to 'involve trainees whilst modelling a process of facilitating throughout their training' (Mckenzie-Mavinga 2005: 298). She also 'engaged colleagues in integrating workshops on black issues into the counsellor training curriculum'. Isha Mckenzie-Mavinga (2005: 298) continues:

Two main concepts emerged from the study process: Firstly, the concept of 'Finding a Voice', which portrays the 'emancipatory' (Denzin, 1989) process evolving from the silence of not having previously had dialogue about black issues within training programmes. ... As a staff team we recognised that trainees' understanding could be supported by providing a space to complement racism. The second concept which emerged from the study process, 'Recognition Trauma', has been applied to the fear experienced by both black and white trainees when they become fully conscious of the impact of racism on their lives; for example, in their narratives white trainees expressed feelings of guilt and fear when they listened to black trainees' experiences and feelings about racism; black trainees experienced powerful feelings about being victims of racism and their process of internalising oppression. These recognition traumas appeared to create stuckness and a perceived lack of safety to explore on a deeper level.

Isha's dual role as trainer and researcher triggered some special ethical considerations, as we explored earlier in Chapter 7 on ethics. Her approach illustrates a not uncommon dilemma in practice-based research in terms of the enmeshed insider perspective.

Co-operative inquiry into school-based therapy

Another example of collaborative research that is also positioned in education is the research by Stephen Adams-Langley (2011: 135), mentioned earlier, about school-based therapy.

> This final project has sought to bring alive the voices and qualitative experience of the key players in the service, and rather than present evidence-based practice, present the narrative of practice-based evidence, through qualitative inquiry and field-based exploration and explanation.

Stephen has managed Place2Be services in Nottingham, Medway and Cardiff as well as Enfield, Lambeth and Camden, and chooses to base his research 'in the inner city in London where I have managed the Place2Be programmes for fourteen years'. As mentioned earlier, Stephen shares reflections about his personal and professional investment and how this 'insider' perspective may impact his research. He writes about how he 'was a child from a highly volatile family structure with early and enduring experiences of parental rejection and ambivalence ... with frequent hospitalisations and poor attendance at school leading to isolation, school refusal and academic failure'.

Inductive *and* deductive reasoning

We suggested earlier that methodology 'is more than a set of research methods and a project plan', as Costley et al. (2010: 81, 165) put it, and that 'methodology is about how you, the researcher, see the world'. In Stephen's case, the choice to work with grounded theory, involves an attempt to combine two contrasting 'world-views'. Inductive and deductive reasoning involve different world views and grounded theory embraces the attempt to combine these two different approaches to reality.

Moule and Hek (2011: 57–8) conclude that inductive and deductive reasoning reflects 'more than a way of collecting data; rather, they are an overall commitment within the research process ... inductive and hypothetic-deductive approaches to research should be called methodologies'.

The inductive approach involves making 'sense of them from the individual's perspective', while the focus in deductive reasoning revolves around generalisability and prediction based on what individuals (or things) hold in common. In grounded theory, the researcher 'starts from the ground and works up in an inductive fashion, to make sense of what people say about their experiences, and then convert those statements into theoretical proposition' (Stanley 2006: 65). Moule and Hek (2011: 58) refer to grounded theory in terms of:

> [Grounded theory is] a systematic procedure for developing a theory about a phenomenon from the collected data. As the researcher examines the data, collected by observations or interviews, themes and concepts are identified. The researcher then returns frequently to the data, looking for further evidence of the themes and revising the research question as issues arise from the data. ... In many ways, grounded theory is perceived as the far end of the inductive continuum as theories are actually produced.

Stephen offers an example of the development of an epistemological and methodological stance in the research. He considers his choice of working within the framework of grounded theory.

Case study

The Place to be in the Inner City (Adams-Langley 2011)

As an existential humanistic psychotherapist, I value the phenomenological method to elicit subject meaning and experience, and grounded theory is a qualitative methodology aligned to this world view. I also considered narrative and free association and interview methodology (Hollway and Jefferson 2000), but felt that this would not generate the wide range of data I might expect from grounded theory analysis, employing semi-structured interviews with six participants. (Adams-Langley 2011: 26)

An influencing factor in his choice of theory was Stephen's role as an insider. He was attracted by the way the grounded theory would 'attend to bias and research risk, by emphasising the personal experience as an inevitable factor':

> As an 'insider' researcher, I have to admit my bias in relation to the research question and scope, and the bias of becoming complacent and positivistic, regarding the data from the Place2Be staff ... Strauss and Corbin (2008) attend to this bias and research risk, by emphasising the personal experience as an inevitable factor, and suggest that we use our bias to stimulate thinking about the various properties of the data and dimension of concepts, and indeed this was my experience. They warn that sometimes researchers become so engrossed in their investigations, that they do not realise that they have come to accept the assumptions and beliefs of their respondents.

Grounded theory, continues Stephen, emphasises the importance of stepping 'away from the data and be[ing] surprised by my assumptions and beliefs and that of the participants'. This was something which Stephen wanted to incorporate in the way he aimed to generate knowledge. He is hoping to 'produce a research study of "multiple truths"'.

A grounded researcher must walk a fine line into getting into the hearts and minds of respondents, while keeping enough distance to be able to clarify and analyse the data. Attempting to stay at the conceptual level and keeping a journal of my thoughts, feelings and cognitions helped me to 'step way' from the data and be surprised by my assumptions and beliefs and that of the participants. Strauss and Corbin (2008) refer to 'waving the red flag,' when one is becoming too certain of the data. They are wary of the assumption that a researcher can 'bracket' their beliefs or perspectives. My research journal enabled me to record and process my responses to the emerging data, and my attendant anxiety, to produce a research study of 'multiple truths'. Inevitably we are shaped by as well as shaping of our research.

Stephen incorporates a co-operative inquiry in his research as a means of achieving the important element of 'being surprised' and adopting new and different angles to his 'insider' perspective. The study developed into a three-stage process, which is referred to below in extracts which particularly highlight the collaborative aspect of Stephen's research. His study involved:

- Interviewing six head teachers (grounded theory: Strauss and Corbin 2008)

Following my write up of the head teacher interviews, I sent all six head teachers my draft and asked for their comments and perspectives. The aim was to verify the accuracy and tone of the account from the participants, and be open to challenge and disagreement or validation. (Adams-Langley 2011: 82)

- Establishing a co-operative inquiry group with ten participant senior Place2Be school project managers

Stephen (Adams-Langley 2011: 88) describes the group in terms of a group to do research with rather than on:

The co-operative inquiry group ... was comprised of ten experienced school project managers, a parent worker and a hub manager. I had sent the twelve members of the group a paper explaining the principle of a co-operative inquiry group

(Heron 1996; Reason 1994) ... and a consent letter. ... The one and a half hour meeting was taped and later transcribed, although all participants were offered confidentiality and anonymity for their contribution. I started the meeting by intro-ducing to the group my motivation for undertaking the practitioner doctorate. ... I then explained my role to the group to attempt to facilitate a learning environ-ment, and to draw on the considerable skills, experience and insights of the group. I reflected on my intention to conduct research with people, rather than on them. ... This is particularly critical in my approach to the two case studies, which will involve children and parents, and where I will need to be alert to the sensitivity and ethical issues of the child and parent co-operation, in this phase of the research. ... I requested help in reflecting upon the following issues:

- How to structure interviews with head teachers and questions on topics of inquiry in this phase.
- Identifying 'hard to reach' children for case study research in spring and sum-mer 2011, with a random selection within the group, of two referrals from a potential of twelve. Each participant to refer one child, and we will pick the name out of the hat, subject to parental and child consent, with a waiting list of children, in the event of negative consent.
- The commitment from the whole group to emotional honesty and experiential inquiry, based on critical subjectivity and collaboration.
- In the first reflective phase of the group, we would reflect on the experience of being school-based therapists, and I would draw on my previous research account and interviews with six school project managers.

My role in the group was to facilitate questions, ideas and propositions about the inquiry and focus of the research. I would endeavour to facilitate the process and content of inquiry, by taping all the meetings and analysing content, reflect[ing] on the psychological process, writ[ing] up the account, and present[ing] to the group by e-mail in advance, on subsequent co-operative inquiry group meetings within the next six months. I would record any discrepancies or disagreements in my written account, and hope to facilitate mutual growth, participation and skills for participants of the group, rooted in subjective emotional awareness and feed-back. (Adams-Langley 2011: 88)

Activity

Co-operative research

Identify five or six people who can contribute to your research. Other therapists? Colleagues at work?

The examples below illustrate how Stephen approached and explained to the participants about the co-operative inquiry group. Read Stephen's consent letter and the information about co-operative inquiry, and think of a context where you could apply this approach to your own research.

Example of consent letter for co-operative inquiry group (Adams-Langley 2011)

1st September 2010

Dear Colleagues,

Thank you for your agreement to participate in a co-operative inquiry group to consider the following topic in a doctoral research study:

'The Place2Be in the inner city primary school: How can a voluntary sector mental health service have an impact on children's mental health and the school environment?'

An information sheet about co-operative inquiry (Heron, 1996; Reason, 1994) is attached to this letter to explain the research method and introduce some key ideas.

Ethical research is undertaken with people, not on them, and for such an important research into school-based child mental health, I believe the quality and impact of the doctoral research dissertation and products will be considerably enhanced and more truthful and interesting to read with the co-operation of the group. I would value your insights and ideas in the course of several meetings over the next 12 months at a primary school. Our first meeting has been arranged for the .... at 9:30 a.m. for one hour. I will tape and then transcribe the responses of the group which will help to consider the interviews with head teachers and children and parent involvement in the research.

All responses will be entirely confidential and anonymous, and you or your contribution will not be identified in the final paper.

I do intend to publish products of this doctoral research with the exception of the two child case studies, which I feel would be unethical and uncomfortable.

I look forward to meeting with you all and introducing the principles and practice of co-operative inquiry.

Yours sincerely

S.J. Adams-Langley, Regional Manager

I do / do not consent to be part of a co-operative inquiry group for the purpose of the doctoral research study.

Name...................................... Date...........................

Information for Co-operative Inquiry Group
Co-operative inquiry (Heron 1996; Reason 1994)

Research into the human condition

- each person is co-subject and co-researcher in the reflection phase;
- possibility of reciprocal participative knowing;
- participative decision-making and reflectivity;
- knowing is mutual awakening – mutual participative awareness;
- recent work on emotional intelligence shows that effective choice is rooted in emotional values;
- co-operative inquiry does research **with** people, not on them;
- content and method are reflected upon by all research participants in the group;
- the full range of human sensibilities is available as an instrument of inquiry;
- the researcher's account of the subjects' perspectives is validated and checked with the subjects themselves.

First reflection phase

- topic of the inquiry and launching statement;
- interviewing six head teachers on the value of The Place2Be and the impact of the school-based mental health service in their school;
- scope of the interview;
- areas of inquiry;
- contract with the group;
- collaboration – data recorded, written up and sent to all members of group, in advance;
- shared learning will comprise four to six meetings of one hour;
- this will be recorded on a tape machine and analysed by researcher (SAL);
- objectivity is a figment of our minds (Reason 1994);
- the validity of our encounter with experience rests on high-quality, critical, self-aware, discriminating and informed judgements of the co-researchers;
- vulnerability of openness can lead to experiential inquiry based on integrity and critical subjectivity;
- co-operative inquiry is an emergent process.

(Continued)

(Continued)

For whom is this research?

- The Place2Be;
- advance the argument for school-based mental health;
- research and advisory group;
- Place2Reflect;
- co-operative inquiry – group mutual participation – insight and growth – awareness;
- policies and procedures to train and support new colleagues, in new schools and new hubs.

My role within the group

- to facilitate questions, ideas and propositions about the inquiry and focus of research;
- to facilitate process and content of inquiry, by taping all the meetings and analysing content, writing up and presenting content back to the group, for further reflection and challenge;
- to support the group in expressing intuitive and tacit knowing and facilitating propositional knowledge.

If you have a question or query that you feel would be difficult to raise with me, you can speak to Mr xxxx xxxx, Chair of xxxxx. Telephone: xxxxxx.

Figure 13.3   Co-operative inquiry, Information sheet (Adams-Langley 2011)

Engaging with the 'other'

We looked earlier at Qualley's (1997) definition of reflexivity in terms of 'engaging with the other'. Stephen's research process illustrates this on different levels. He refers, to start with, to all his participants as 'highly engaged and committed individuals'. It is clear that both the one-to-one interviews and the co-operative inquiry group had a 'profound impact' upon him. Stephen (Adams-Langley 2011: 56) writes:

> The emotional intensity in the one-to-one interviews and group meeting had a profound impact upon me as a researcher. ... The group focus interview was significant in raising my awareness to the lack of attention paid in the initial interviews to

the emotional responses of the participants, to the task of providing a counselling service to children in the complex system of a primary school. ... One participant stated that: 'I couldn't engage with the first part of the paper, it seemed rather dry and boring...'. ... This was a challenge that was direct and revelatory in that in my anxiety as a novice researcher I had stayed primarily at the cognitive level, and my questions to participants shaped their cognitive responses.

Stephen (Adams-Langley 2011: 63) continues to reflect over the impact of the feedback regarding his report being 'dry':

I became aware that my anxiety as a researcher had paralysed my 'voice', and that the rigidity and dryness which is reflected in the grounded theory categories is an accurate reflection of my cognitive bias at this stage of the research. I entered the research with two left feet in lead boots due to my anxiety, and therefore felt unable to dance and move with the participants in the first round of interviews. I felt that the participants intuitively recognised this anxiety and we were able to 'dance together' in the group co-operative inquiry in a clumsy, but more authentic manner.

To further secure ongoing and challenging feedback Stephen reflects in his dissertation to reading and discussing arts exhibitions and attending seminars, and sometimes these took Stephen out of his comfort zone:

I was intrigued by Els van Ooijen's seminar on 'Research as a Vehicle for Personal and Professional Integration', and prepared for the seminar by reading her paper on 'The Magic Crystal: A Search for Integration', and considering her experience of the 'paradigm shift' in my own journey. *Initially I found the process of emerging from behind the researcher 'curtain' as quite painful and challenging, and the paradigm shift for me was to place myself as a practitioner-researcher at the heart of my research.* I hoped that this would result in a more ethical, truthful and interesting product. ... Els discussed the ethical implications of inviting the client to see what has been written about them as 'fair and ethical', and this was another key impact on my research through my attendance at this seminar. I intend to show the case studies to the parents and therapists and send the grounded theory analysis of head teacher interviews and experience back to them for comment and potential challenge. This is what I believed Els was promoting through ... the ethic of care which can be found in Rogers, and phenomenological research and philosophy. Els discussed the 'heuristic swamp', and the need for inter-subjectivity and critical friends in research. I hope my case studies are a reflection of self inquiry with others rather on them, with a direct challenge to the dubious attempt to remain obscure or hidden behind the 'research curtain'.

Like in the previous example with Pamela Stewart's prison-based research, an essential aspect is to capture the surrounding atmosphere. Stephen writes about aiming for that when 'the interviews with the head teachers, gave a "voice" to the realities and the pressure of living in deprived parts of inner city London':

> I interviewed one head teacher in a school, and walked through an estate to reach the primary school. The walk ways and stair wells were littered with debris, rubbish bags spilling contents, used nappies and used syringes and needles as the stair wells are often used as 'shooting galleries' by heroin users. *The squalor and oppressive atmosphere can hardly be described, and I felt a rising anger at the conditions to which so many children and families are expected to accept.* As a former community worker in the area fifteen years ago, I was aware of the infestation of cockroaches and pharaoh ants in the majority of flats on the estate and how intimidating the area can appear at night. If Disraeli described Victorian Britain as 'two nations' of rich and poor, one hundred years later there is certainly 'two cities' in London, dividing the rich and poor citizens and their children. ...
>
> My sense of many of the inner city schools was that of 'pressure cookers', where head teachers and their staff have the challenging task of managing government and local authority targets, attend to volatile dynamics between children, and support parents where the pressures of poverty, deprivation and domestic violence place a heavy psychological burden on head teachers, who are more often trusted by parents, rather than social services, where the threshold for support is under increasing pressure. ...
>
> In three interviews I was kept waiting by the head teacher, since in two cases, head teachers had serious child protection cases which took priority. In the third interview, the head teacher had to leave half way through as a physical conflict between two students required his practical support of a class room teacher. We were able to convene one hour later and complete the interview ...
>
> *My reflexive response* to the interviews was one of feeling the pressures on head teachers.

Stephen illustrates the role of practitioner researchers in terms of 'telling it as it is', in terms of capturing the complexities involved in the reality that he aims to research. He includes reflections around how the research impacts him personally. Stephen (Adams-Langley 2011: 90) ponders, for instance, over how the feedback of the co-operative inquiry group had left him feeling 'raw and vulnerable' after tapping into the uncomfortable recognition of his own childhood experience of physical and emotional abuse:

> My own reflection, after I had listened to the tape of the group was that I was struggling with the return to 'feeling' the work, and the uncomfortable recognition of my own situation and childhood experience of physical and emotional

abuse. At this stage of the doctorate, I am feeling raw and exposed, and feeling flooded with my own experience as a child, which has been provoked by the co-operative inquiry group, and the emotional honesty and the engagement of the members and myself.

Put into the context of the theoretical framework for his study, Stephen explores his own reaction within the framework for co-operative inquiry theory, and with reference to Heron (1996) and Reason (1994):

Heron (1996) refers to the empathy, harmonic resonance and receptivity which are present in the co-operative inquiry group, and I feel the identification and attunement with the group has touched upon my childhood experience and human sensibility, which I have repressed, for many years, due to the demands of a challenging work role and my own survival mechanism. I shall need to ensure that the wounded helper in me is acknowledged and supported. Reason (1994) makes reference to this emotional identification and openness as the 'touch stone of the inquiry method' (Reason, 1994: 43). This phase of the group involves experiential knowing, such that superficial understandings are elaborated and developed through immersion and creative insights. He makes reference to critical subjectivity and the resonance with being, whereby we can experience presences in our world, by attunement, resonance and empathy, in direct acquaintance and encounter. The emotional honesty of the group, and the resonance with the experience of children, returns myself and the group to the conscious use of imagination and memory in co-operative inquiry.

Stephen (Adams-Langley 2011: 80–88) refers to the data analysis as pains-takingly labour intensive. The extract below illustrates how the coding process resulted in categories ranging from 'the mental health needs of children and parents' to 'the strengths of the Place2Be school mental health service':

The interviews were analysed using grounded theory methodology (Strauss and Corbin 2008) .... The intention in this methodology is to identify recurring meaning categories across interviews using a method of open coding and constant comparison. The aim is to create a description and theory from the data itself rather than fitting the data into an external model. The theory generated is thus grounded in the data (Strauss and Corbin 2008). To attempt to retain the voice of the participants, analysis of interview material was made directly from the audio recordings instead of from written transcripts. There is synchronisation of data

(Continued)

(Continued)

collection and analysis, and I analysed the data as soon as possible following the interview so that I could become more sensitised to the issues and areas within the emerging theoretical framework. The data from each interview was coded in a three-stage process ....

Categories were built up from 445 meaning units in the transcripts. The meaning units were ascribed to more than one category, as appropriate. Categories were systematically related and developed as some initial categories became subsumed by others, resulting in seven main categories. These categories cover the mental health needs of children and parents, children who were identified by participants as 'hard to reach' and a category examining the accessibility of the mental health service. Further categories include: the barriers to therapeutic efficacy, the characteristics of the Place2Be school project manager, measuring the impact of the therapeutic intervention, and the strengths of the Place2Be school mental health service, before considering the implications of the data for clinical practice and service delivery.

Below is an extract from the first category that Stephen Adams-Langley (2011: 86–88) identifies through the grounded theory method.

Case study

(Data analysis of interviews (Adams-Langley 2011: 86))

Category one: Mental health needs of children and parents

The six participants all identified socio-economic deprivation of children and parents as linked to the mental health risks of children and families. Overcrowding in small flats on council estates with high rates of crime were identified in creating pressure and a climate of fear and psycho-social pressure for children and parents. Temporary housing and inadequate emergency accommodation were a common occurrence for children in the cluster of primary schools. Absent or violent fathers and relatively high levels of abuse in the form of neglect, emotional abuse or harsh physical abuse were identified as leading to depression and anxiety for children, who were referred to the Place2Be. Participants felt that children were often exposed to domestic violence in the home, which was exacerbated by parent's use of drugs and alcohol. In one school, the school project manager estimated that 90% of the children were from West African cultures where parents were seeking asylum, and some had failed their application for asylum and were 'in hiding'. ...

Category eight: Impact on school staff

Interview analysis (Adams-Langley 2011: 88)

The impact on school staff had been considerable in all the schools, with participants reflecting on how they and their school staff have become more nurturing of the children, and emotionally aware, as the impact of the school based mental health service had helped change the culture towards children and children's emotional and mental well-being. ...

...participants described the loss of the Place2Be service as 'devastating' or 'unthinkable'. ... "My teachers can now teach" was a reflection by several head teachers, who also reflected on the impact of the service in helping them develop an emotionally literate and calmer school.

In an extract from his final chapter, some of the overall outcome of the study is described as follows:

The grounded theory analysis of six head teachers and six school project managers also revealed The Place2Be has considerable impact on the school environment. The Place2Think provided psychological consultation for teachers, to enable them to interpret, understand and tolerate children's challenging and sometimes inexplicable behaviour. ... The Place2Be provided 'strategies for coping', which head teachers felt calmed the challenges of both the classroom and aggression in the playground. Head teachers reported that the school project manager was a trusted member of their team, who was immediately available and offered a different perspective on understanding and managing the behaviour of a complex child with multiple needs. The lowering of disruption and aggression was noted by the majority of the head teachers and was consequently highly valued. As one participant noted, 'my teachers can now teach' (Head teacher). ... The school environment was also improved, with head teachers reporting that emotional literacy, emotional well-being and therapeutic ethos was increasingly part of their school culture, as Place2Be had an impact on staff attitudes, to some acting out and challenging children and children who were vulnerable, bullied, excluded from friendships, withdrawn, depressed or disengaged with education tasks and attainment.

Recommended reading

Livholts, M. (ed.) (2013) *Emergent Writing Methodologies in Feminist Studies.* London: Routledge.

This edited collection focuses on the emergence of writing methodologies in feminist studies and their implications for the study of power and change.

FOURTEEN   Making an impact

Simon du Plock

Simon du Plock writes about the impact of research and discusses some of the ways of communicating our research findings with the outside world.

- Doctoral research journeys
- PhD thesis
- Professional doctorates
- Products
- Stakeholder
- Existential crisis
- Passionate engagement
- Outcome
- Demonstrating impact
- Systematic inquiry
- Change
- Reflexive evaluation
- Pluralism
- Bibliotherapy

Impact: The force or action of one object hitting another; a powerful effect which something, especially something new, has on a situation or person.

(Definition of 'impact' (noun), *Cambridge Advanced Learner's Dictionary and Thesaurus*)

Discussion of doctoral level research in the arts and the humanities has rarely included significant focus on how research findings will be communicated to the world beyond the university, and dissemination is often given scant attention in the traditional PhD thesis. PhD candidates tend to include some brief indications of the further research which may be indicated by their work (often with the object of paving the way for post-doctoral research), but they do not ordinarily set out a detailed strategy which will enable their research findings to make a difference to the world beyond the academy. This may, in part, be a legacy of the traditional role of the PhD to act as a vehicle for the candidate to demonstrate their fitness to join the academic research community. As the UK Council for Graduate Education (UK Council for Graduate Education 2002: 11) notes:

> In the latter half of the twentieth century, there was a major change in the pub-
> lic attitude to Research in Universities. Research has come to be seen as the
> defining characteristic of academics, so that it has become almost impossible
> in most universities for academics to be appointed without having first com-
> pleted a PhD. Possession of a PhD establishes a minimum level of capability in
> research which is generally a necessary, although certainly not sufficient, condi-
> tion for appointment to an academic position.

Mullins and Kiley (2002: 380), in a detailed analysis of the factors which a sample of thirty assessors take into account when examining a PhD, found that they 'were looking for students who exhibited a sense of confidence in the way they dealt with the material and a level of sophistication in the way they presented their argument'. This approach suggests that assessors continue to be primarily concerned with the degree to which a student is able to defend their 'thesis' – in the sense of a statement or theory that is put forward as a premise to be maintained or proved. They did not find that examiners identified a discussion of impact as a necessary component of a thesis; rather, the thesis appears to be viewed as a discrete entity.

A good thesis is one which demonstrates 'scholarship', defined as evi-dence of originality, coherence, and the autonomy and independence of the student. Perhaps surprisingly, only half of the assessors in Mullins and Kiley's study stated they were influenced positively if a candidate's work had been accepted for publication in a reputable journal – one of the key ways in which their work might reach a wider audience and begin to make an impact.

The great expansion of higher education and the concomitant develop-ment of a wide range of doctorates beyond the standard PhD model, espe-cially over the past quarter century, means that research students are increasingly expected to evidence the wider relevance of their work. The growth of Professional Doctorates, for example, has led to a gradual move away from a concern with knowledge-based research, and a greater focus on research into the nature of professional practice. This is congruent with the rationale for such doctorates (UK Council for Graduate Education 2002: 34):

> One of the main driving forces behind the development of Professional
> Doctorates is the view that there is a need for a research based approach to
> deal with some of the complex problems faced by various professions. The
> research element is therefore usually carried out in a professional context, and
> in a way which is relevant to the needs of the individual candidate and his/her
> employing organisation.

I first entered the world of doctoral research over twenty years ago when, after a period working as a research officer in a provincial university, I applied to a world-famous institution to undertake a Master's degree in industrial relations. In my previous research role I had been the junior member in a small team of sociologists investigating the socialisation of new recruits into the culture of a police training college, and I envisaged that my Master's dissertation would be an extension of some aspects of this. To my surprise, I was invited to compete for one of the four-year PhD research scholarships maintained by this prestigious university, and I was delighted to be successful. There was one caveat, though, and that was the large one that I should research patterns of union and professional organisation membership among NHS nurses, and that I would do this using the university's renowned computer systems. Flushed with the excitement of winning a scholarship, I immediately agreed and put my own broadly qualitative research interests to one side. At the time I reasoned that I had nothing to lose by complying with the research focus of my new university, and everything to gain since their PhD would certainly give me a greatly enhanced access to academic posts in the future. While I did not formulate it in the language of impact at the time, my reasoning was that a connection with this institution would enable me to re-enter academia at a level where I would be able to make a worthwhile difference to professional practice.

Reflecting on this now, I can see that in allowing myself to be seduced into a research topic which held little intrinsic interest for me I had, in fact, relinquished the opportunity to advance in a field – sociology of deviancy – with which I had been fascinated for some time; rather than take what promised to be a fast lane to an academic post, I had consigned myself to an extended period wandering the byways of industrial psychology. Nearly three years later, and with a date set for the final viva, I realised I could not continue down this road. Looking back at the research journal notes which I still have, I find frequent rumination on the meaninglessness of the research for me: what, I asked, was the *use* of the hundreds of pages of statistical analysis I had compiled? Would anyone else ever read it? And if even they did, what would they *do* with it? Finally, very late one night, and in the throes of what I now understand to be an existential crisis, I shredded as much of the material as I could and disposed of the remainder down the communal rubbish chute of the tower block where I lived. Early next morning I let myself into the computer lab and wiped all the records clean. I still remember the feeling of elation and liberation this brought.

It might seem self-indulgent to recount this experience, but my reason for doing so is to bring what we mean by 'impact', and its significance, into sharper focus. I look back on this episode of my life with a sense of achievement because it was one in which I gained an enhanced sense of what was important for me both personally and professionally. While the outcome was quite different from that which I had expected, my doctoral work had a very significant impact on me: I discovered, or re-discovered, my values and learned that I did not want to devote the very considerable time and energy required for doctoral research to something which was not genuinely of pressing concern to me. That it was *possible* for me to do so was evident from the three years I had spent in this endeavour, but rigorous reflection had led me to the conclusion that I work most effectively when I feel passionately engaged with my topic. I often ask new candidates to the research doctorate I currently lead to think carefully and take the time to arrive at a topic which is of genuine interest to them, rather than hurriedly grasp at something second-hand. In many respects, I feel that the best doctoral project is something which the candidate would be motivated to pursue even if they were not enrolled on a doctoral programme. The programme provides a structure for the research journey, but the candidate might have undertaken it in some form or other regardless.

Activity

This exercise is designed to help you identify the significance of your research *to you*, and to think about whether you are likely to be able to pursue it most effectively inside the structure of a doctoral programme, or by taking an independent route.

Imagine that you are at the beginning of a doctoral research journey. Take a few minutes to think about a topic on which you might wish to conduct a piece of research. Note down what comes to mind in relation to the following questions:

- If you have already begun to explore this particular topic prior to embarking on a doctorate, how have you done so?
- What originally motivated you to explore this topic, and what motivates you now? Does being on a doctorate lead you to feel more motivated about your project, and if so, can you explore this?
- How does being a doctoral candidate assist you to engage with others in the field? Are there any ways in which being on a doctoral programme might make it more difficult for you to pursue your exploration?
- What were your thoughts about how you might engage with stakeholders to encourage changes to professional practice in this area?
- Imagine for a moment that for some reason you were not able to continue on the doctorate. What would be the consequences for your research? If you were to continue with a project, what form would it take and in what ways might it be different? Might you feel unable to progress some aspects of your research? Might you feel free to look at others in ways which do not seem appropriate for a doctorate?
- Finally, what do you feel the personal and professional impact of doctoral research might be for you?

So how *can* the doctoral researcher, particularly the researcher exploring an aspect of therapy, make an impact? And, given that they are intent on earning a doctoral award, how can they *demonstrate* this impact? The first thing to say is that for their project to impact upon the wider therapy provider and therapy-consuming communities it must be communicated to these potentially interested parties, and it must, if it is to be adopted by them, be in some genuine respect *useful*. Research should be actively defined as inclusive of communication of the results if it is to be viewed as research at all, rather than as a form of personal learning generation. As McLeod (2001: 4) argues:

> A useful working definition of research is: a systematic process of critical inquiry leading to valid propositions and conclusions that are communicated to interested others.

In other words, research is not a private activity – it has to get out into the world if it is to count for anything. In this sense, the myriad of Master's dissertations and Doctoral theses which sit unread on library shelves or in electronic archives may be thought of as only *technically* research.

It is worth emphasising that a project's potential for impact is very often lessened by the wrong choice of method for the researcher's target audience, or by the pursuit of the wrong question. Researchers are well advised to begin by asking themselves what exactly it is that they want to change, who the powerful stakeholders are in relation to this possible change, and who therefore they need to communicate with. Only then is it sensible to decide upon a particular methodology. Examples abound of therapy research projects that did not make an impact because they did not utilise the methodology preferred by those the researcher set out to influence. Elliott (2002) refers to this phenomenon as 'rendering unto Caesar that which is Caesar's' – the coin of the realm being what the realm values. Researchers need to think strategically about the way they engage with stakeholders, and understand how different stakeholders can be addressed successfully. So it is that random control trials (RCTs) influence policy makers because they are concerned with general effects across a whole population. Given their focus, it is hardly surprising that this is the case, and there is little point in bemoaning that they are not more interested in, for example, the small qualitative enquiries which we, as qualitatively-minded researchers, most value.

The same is generally true of commissioners of services in commercial environments: an Employee Assistance Programme (EAP), for example, is required to demonstrate its worth in terms of its beneficial impact on the finances of the company through a reduction in absenteeism or economies in managing redundancies. Other perspectives will require different methodologies: practitioners, for example, have relatively little interest in RCTs or statistics (and may occasionally even feel quite negative about them), but they can be readily engaged via qualitative investigations of the experience of individuals from groups of interest, such as specific client populations. Clients typically are most exercised by the headline results of RCTs (since they want to know 'will this work for someone like me?'), and then want information about what the experience of being a client will be like (and so are interested in short and jargon-free individual accounts).

Any study will benefit from a reflexive evaluation of itself to regularly review the extent to which the chosen methodology is fit for purpose. While a study made sense to a researcher and their supervisor, this does not necessarily mean that others will pay attention to it. Whoever the researcher wants to influence, their study must have some practical utility. It is helpful to think about utility as the ultimate arbiter of methodological choice: if your audience will not find it useful, why are you doing it? *What* use will they make of it; indeed, what *sense* will they be able to make of it? Not only does the researcher need to identify key stakeholders, understand their perspective and requirements in depth and then design methods to fit their interests, but they also need to write up their work in a way which will enable their audience to make the fullest use of their findings. Typically, managers will demand brief, statistically convincing (but simple) summaries; counsellors want quotes and vivid insights; clients want to know proposed treatments and procedures are safe, and they want to be able to read vignettes of other clients' experience.

Beyond this, and of great importance in terms of dissemination, researchers should ensure that they use appropriate and effective routes to reach their audiences. Since few clients actively seek out information, the researcher needs to think about where and in what form information can be made available: attractive posters on GP surgery notice boards, for example, might encourage clients to explore further on the internet. Innovative researchers might want to cast their net more widely in order to engage clients in other places they regularly frequent. Therapists tend to be very busy people, who are more likely to be engaged via professional journals such as *The Psychologist*, *The Psychotherapist* and *Therapy Today*, rather than specialist peer-reviewed research journals, and they can also be reached via conferences and continuous professional development (CPD) events. While publication in peer-reviewed journals remains the key to establishing the validity of a research project (and even here care needs to be taken to publish in the most appropriate journal as some are more prestigious than others and attract an international readership), readership per paper will always be relatively low. If we are serious about making an impact we need to think beyond the standard academic media to commissioned writing for newspapers and popular magazines. Publication here can have a disproportionate impact. For many years, the British Association for Counselling and Psychotherapy (BACP) strategy for influencing attitudes to counselling among the general public centred on women's magazines which, while low-status professionally speaking, reached a receptive audience and so constituted a significant influence on a group (women) who would themselves be influential.

My colleague, Dr Stephen Goss, recounts how he was able, via his own PhD research and a series of papers, to address specifically the concerns of a range of EAP stakeholders. Goss, S. P. and Mearns, D. (1997) 'Applied pluralism in the evaluation of employee counselling' appeared in the *British Journal of Guidance and Counselling* and was, as he explains:

> ...a deliberate attempt to have an impact on several audiences and so included financial impact from observable behaviour change, psychometric recording of change to convince my fellow academic psychology researchers, goal attainment measures to speak to clients about how far people have their needs met and qualitative accounts of experience from multiple perspectives. This influenced teaching bodies who wanted to hear that support for teachers was both needed and effective so this paper in a specialist location led directly to work on the economic impact of providing counselling for all teachers funded by the Teacher's Benevolent Fund which showed potential savings of tens of millions, which would pay for a lot of counselling. That was preceded by an early report on teacher stress and the possible role of counselling in the Times Ed in 1995 which laid the groundwork for the topic to become 'hot' and afterwards led to a commissioned specialist report (Goss, S.P. (2002) *Counselling: A Quiet Revolution*. London: Teacher's Benevolent Fund) that was circulated directly to all LEAs, the Department of Education, MPs, Ministers, and all head teachers in the UK. There was also a planned campaign of conference presentations (counselling and education fields) and papers in specialist journals and magazines. End result is that all teachers in Scotland now have at least theoretical access to counselling for work-related issues. Teachers accept it because they know what they will get; head teachers accept it because they were shown that their staff will be more effective and less stressed so their jobs will be easier; counsellors accept it because they understand how the process works and what the important features of service provision in that field are; managers accept paying for it because they know it pays off for them in the longer term by reducing absenteeism/presenteeism and so on; policy makers accept it because the economic arguments were very clear indeed and it addressed their concern to reduce budgets and appear to be caring at the same time.

(S.P. Goss, personal email to S. du Plock, 21 December 2012)

PhD researchers in the arts and humanities are, though, rarely expected to function as change agents who craft careful strategies aimed at making an impact on their field. While they may, and increasingly do, attempt to evidence the relevance of their work for the wider world, this is not normally a requirement for the award of the degree. I finally completed a Practitioner Doctorate in the context of a programme where demonstration of impact was considered integral to research. While undertaking a traditional PhD can have a considerable impact on the researcher, if not on the wider field, the ethos of a Practitioner Doctorate is likely to lead to significant consequences for both. The philosophy at the heart of the Doctorate in Psychotherapy by Professional Practice (DPsych), a joint Middlesex University and Metanoia Institute programme, provides an excellent example of the potential for impact of a Practitioner Doctorate. The DPsych was designed to support fully-qualified professional therapeutic practitioners to update and expand their application of theory, evaluate their own practice and critique their own assumptions with particular attention to current developments and research outcomes in the field – and all while working towards obtaining a doctorate. This activity is not undertaken in isolation (as it is typically in the traditional PhD), but in regular collaboration with other interested parties. Candidates (as these senior practitioners are termed) are required to produce a 'Final Product' – essentially a research and development enterprise as opposed to a research-based thesis. Successful candidates are expected to evidence not only their ability to generate and defend a thesis, but also:

- their professional experience developed continuously through active and effective engagement with individuals and groups of clients in a wide range of contexts;
- the forms of research resulting in 'products' of demonstrable interest and usefulness to practitioners;
- the leadership qualities and skills whereby professionals are able to set up training, consultancy and organisations dedicated to psychotherapy provision.

This focus promotes an ethos of research needing to be useful and active in the world, making a difference and positively influencing the systems in which we work and live.

Activity

Below are some examples of product as they are conceptualised on this Doctorate in Psychotherapy. If you are considering beginning, or are currently undertaking, doctoral research you may find it helpful to think about what you will create in the course of your research.

- Training course manuals with evidence that these courses are already running or commitments by organisations to run them
- Publications, articles, textbooks
- DVDs/videos for distribution to the public and/or professionals
- Evaluated courses
- Establishment of agencies/evaluation of agencies/service providers
- Adoption of the new practices/protocols
- Original/ground-breaking contribution to knowledge and practice.

Your products may be similar or very different, depending on your area of research, the audience for your research, the form any collaboration takes, and the kinds of changes you wish to promote. If you have not already done so, you might like to write your own list, and note how your impact will be evidenced.

I designed my research with the intention of making a contribution to the theory and practice of existential psychotherapy. As an existential therapist myself, I had long been aware of a puzzling discrepancy between the significance this practitioner community accords to existential literature and the extent to which literature of any kind is used in existential therapy itself. The experience of reading literature which explicitly engages with fundamental questions about how to make sense of an essentially meaningless world is frequently a motivation for people to train as existential therapists. Such literature generally features in the curricula of training programmes, yet it seemed that no coherent ideas had been formulated with regard to using this literature as a resource in therapeutic practice.

Clearly a number of stakeholders were involved in this situation, and each of these audiences needed to be engaged in different ways. While Goss devised a strategy to influence practitioners and policy makers in a specific direction, in my own case I decided, if I was to be taken seriously by fellow practitioners, I needed to invite them to come 'inside' the research to collaborate with me. It felt important that my colleagues should understand that my work might offer ways of enriching their therapeutic practice, since at this time very little research had been undertaken by existential therapists and standard texts in the field made almost no reference to its potential value (see, for example, Cooper 2008; Van Deurzen and Arnold-Baker 2005). I initiated this process by identifying a number of key existential practitioners with whom I could begin a dialogue. These practitioners were ideally placed to raise awareness of bibliotherapy in the wider existential community of practice so that when I moved on to the next stage in my strategy, the more formal exploration of this subject via a piece of research, I was inundated by requests from practitioners to be co-researchers.

Accordingly, I undertook a phenomenological research study – as Finlay has noted, 'the existential accent of phenomenological research effortlessly attracts us' (2012: 187) – and communicated my findings via a presentation to an influential group of senior existential therapists, and a paper in a key peer-reviewed journal (du Plock, S. (2005a) '"Silent therapists" and "the community of suffering": some reflections on bibliotherapy from an existential-phenomenological perspective', *Existential Analysis*, 16 (2)). The outcome of this was to bring 'bibliotherapy' into the awareness of existential therapists more fully than before and encourage dialogue within the existential therapy community. I was also concerned to raise awareness among existential counselling psychologists and I did this via a paper on narrative therapy which was published in the BPS Division of Counselling Psychology peer-reviewed journal (du Plock, S. (2005b) 'Some thoughts on the use of narrative approaches in Counselling Psychology', *Counselling Psychology Review*, 20 (2)). This led to an invitation to give the Keynote Address to the 2005 BPS Counselling Psychology Conference, and I took this opportunity to expand on a model of bibliotherapy founded on existential-phenomenological principles. This paper was published the following year in the Division's peer-reviewed journal (du Plock, S. (2006) 'Just what is it that makes contemporary Counselling Psychology so different, so appealing?', *Counselling Psychology Review*, 21 (3)). This helped to increase interest among counselling psychologists inside academia, and led to an invitation to develop an MSc in Narrative Therapy for Roehampton University. I collaborated with Roehampton staff throughout 2006 to pilot this new programme through internal University accreditation. I followed this up in 2007 with a presentation at a key international conference, where I elaborated on this innovative 'Existential Bibliotherapy' (du Plock, S. (2007) 'Using phenomenological research to make a difference: developing a democratic approach to therapeutic reading', *Proceedings of the 25th International Human Science Research Conference, 'New frontiers of phenomenology, beyond postmodernism in empirical research*. Milton Keynes: The Open University). The strategy outlined above indicates how a perceived lack in a practitioner community may be harnessed and form the vehicle for innovations in training which, in turn, can lead to the generation of new models of practice.

While public funding bodies such as the Economic and Social Research Council, in response to cuts in government finance, increasingly require applicants to develop detailed strategies for maximising the impact of their research (see www.esrc.ac.uk/funding-and-guidance/tools-and-resources/impact-toolkit), the majority of recipients are post-doctoral and established researchers. It may well be that, in times of economic austerity and budgetary constraints, a requirement to incorporate an assessment of potential benefits of a doctoral project will eventually become the norm. In this chapter I have argued that there are already excellent reasons for doctoral researchers to take the initiative rather than be driven by economic factors, and show how their work impacts beneficially on therapeutic theory and practice.

Recommended reading

Costley, C., Elliott, G. and Gibbs, P. (2010) *Doing Work-Based Research: Approaches to Enquiry for Insider-Researchers*. London: Sage.

This book addresses key issues in 'insider-research' and is recommended to those who want to deepen their knowledge about work-based learning and practitioner research.

FIFTEEN Concluding remarks

This summary chapter offers some concluding remarks and reflections on the overall content of the book.

- Dialectics
- Reflection
- Dialogue
- Critical engagement
- Pre-conceptions
- Five variants of reflexivity
- Research networks

Typical for practice-based research is its 'situatedness' and that it takes place in offices, hospitals, factories and other 'un-laboratory'-like contexts. It is often conducted by an 'insider'. Practice-based research is, in this sense, never conducted in a vacuum. It has been argued that our interest, methodological approach, critical engagement with literature as well as personal relationships with research participants influence the way we research and will impact the outcome. Rather than seeing subjectivity as an obstacle, reflexivity suggests that we use reflections around our own reactions and experiences as part of the findings. Age, social background, nationality and prior emotional experiences are not only likely to impact the research, as a form of bias, but can also add to the findings. Not dissimilar to the way the therapists bring themselves as persons to explore emotional responses and relationships patterns, researchers invest themselves into the research with an interest in using both their own and others' biases as part of the interesting findings (Figure 15.1).

Based on real-life examples, we have explored different ways of incorporating these influences in our research so that others can access and follow the way they are being integrated in our research. Rupert King, a doctorate

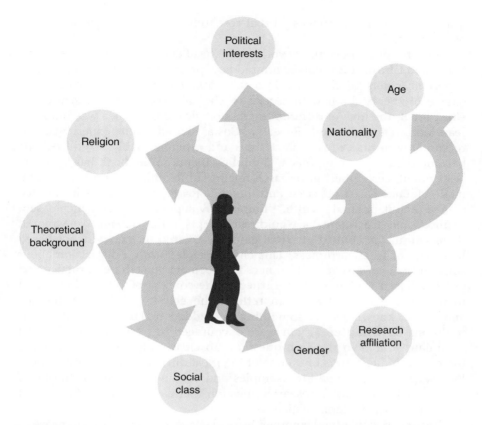

Political
interests

Age

Nationality

Religion

Theoretical
background

Research
affiliation

Gender

Social
class

Figure 15.1 The search for bias (drawing by Finbar Charleson)

in psychotherapy, captures the research experience well. He refers to research as an 'opportunity to understand and creatively develop concepts, which had been themes in my work for some time' and considers his over-all learning experience in terms of 'a series of dialectics':

> What have I learnt from this experience? The initial period of stimulation, crea-tive thinking and exploration was an essential part of the process. But so too was a period of analysis, reflection and dialogue. In short, I struggled with a series of dialectics: (knowing – not-knowing), (self – others), (images – words) and (creativity – analytical thinking). Trying to make sense of these while holding the tension that arose from them was a complex skill I learnt to appreciate.

The aim of this book has been to explore these series of dialectics with the help of real-life examples. Practice-based research is a broad concept. In **Chapter 1**, some of the key characteristics of practitioner research were introduced and explored. We looked, for instance, at 'private' and 'public' research and suggested that research already is a significant part of your life.

The concept of 'personal development' has been a guiding theme in this book, and **Chapter 2** revolved around how prior personal and professional experiences may be integrated into our work. This includes looking at our choice of theory, both with regard to clinical practice and research. In **Chapter 3**, the idea of different methodological approaches was pursued. Jean-Marc Dewaele and Beverley Costa shared their experiences of researching in under-researched areas and explained why mixed methods became their chosen approach. A guiding theme in the book has been the issue about 'certainties' in research relating to the mind. **Chapter 4** examined evidence-based research and the shift towards certainties in the discourse about mental health. 'Empirically-supported', 'evidence-based' methods and 'treatments' are guiding concepts in this debate. We explored them within the context of NICE guidelines based on the evidence-based hierarchy of trustworthiness. This chapter ended with a discussion about some of the overlaps and differences between evidence-based practice and practice-based evidence. We returned to the concept of 'situatedness' and to how practice-based research reflects the activity of routine practice and views knowledge as something embedded in language, culture or traditions. In **Chapter 5**, you were encouraged to begin to consider and formulate your own research question. To clearly identify and articulate the research question is often one of the most difficult aspects of research. We looked at some real-life examples and considered some of the basic aspects of formulating a research question that captures an audience and does your research topic justice.

Chapter 6 concerned another critical stage of the research process, namely the literature review. What else is written in the field? How does your research fit into the existing literature? Professor Simon du Plock explained the essence of 'doing a literature review' and reminded us about how the research question often only becomes defined during this stage, as we engage critically with literature and other ongoing research in your field. Another characteristic of practice-based relationships is the egalitarian and often typically close nature of research relationships. **Chapter 7** concentrated on ethical considerations, with a focus on how the practice-based researcher balances an insider and an outsider role. While close relationships between the researcher and research participants will enhance a rapport and enrich the research findings, the outcome of these collaborative inquiries will invariably often cause surprises – both on a personal and an organisational level. The egalitarian relationships which characterise practice-based research will need to be carefully negotiated. In this chapter, we looked at some differences and overlaps between researcher–participant and therapist–client relationships and considered ways to prepare for the personal change and growth which both types of relationship can spawn.

The concept of 'evidence' is explored from different angles in this book. The meaning of the word 'evidence', as defined in the dictionary, is 'ground for belief or disbelief' (McLeod 1987: 384). **Chapter 8** revolved around belief systems with regard to what we call 'real' in the context of the mind. We considered, for instance, the meaning and impact of epistemology and methodology. Epistemology refers to the theory of knowledge. We looked deeper into how different frameworks of understanding have developed, and how they may impact on the research process and its outcome. Realism, Idealism and postmodern critique were some of the key themes, which were linked to the role of subjectivity in research.

In **Chapter 9**, we returned to the consequences of the inevitable 'messiness' of real-life as opposed to laboratory-based research. Practice-based research is never conducted in a vacuum; it is conducted in busy environments and often in collaboration with many others. While theoretical 'preconceptions' and framings are expected to be considered and explored, the role that personal and socio-cultural pre-understandings and preconceptions may play is still a relatively unexplored area. Freud contended that none of us can claim to be 'masters in our own house'. This assumption is reflected in the argument for reflexive awareness. Reflexivity has been defined with reference to Qualley's (1997) idea about 'engaging with the other', be it with contrasting ideas presented by other researchers, research participants, colleagues, supervisors or 'another part of one's self' (Qualley 1997: 8). Underlying personal and cultural expectations, values and beliefs are held by both the researcher and research participants and will become part of the research. As Qualley (1997: 41) puts it: 'Reflexivity involves a commitment to attending to what we believe, think, and feel while examining how we came to hold those beliefs, thoughts, and feelings.'

We have looked at how implicit, explicit, conscious and unconscious aspects are becoming part of the research process and outcomes, as highlighted in Figure 15.2.

In **Chapter 10**, particular attention was paid to what Finlay and Gough (2003) refer to as the 'five variants' of reflexivity. These variants include reflexivity on introspection, intersubjectivity and mutual collaboration, and reflexivity through social critique and ironic deconstruction. With a specific focus on the research relationships and the impact that both past and present relationships can have on the research, three 'variants' were being explored in more depth. **Chapter 11** looked at examples of reflexivity on introspection as adopted by therapists within humanistic frameworks, adhering to heuristic and autoethnographic approaches in their research. **Chapter 12** focused on reflexivity with an emphasis on intersubjective processes and reflections. We looked at reflexive awareness with attention to 'unconscious' processes, and where both researcher and research participants are explored as 'defended' subjects (Hollway and Jefferson 2000). 'Free association' interviews and the infant-observation

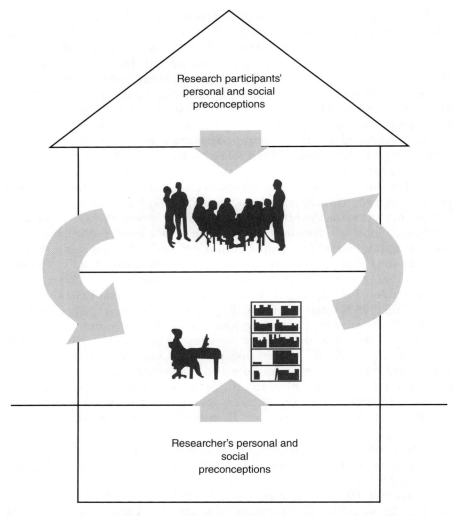

Figure 15.2 Theoretical frameworks, critical engagement with other research, together with underlying personal and cultural values and beliefs held by both the researcher and research participants, feed into and become parts of the research (drawing by Finbar Charleson)

model were offered as examples of reflexive approaches where transference and countertransference play a role in the research. **Chapter 13** addressed a more systemic approach to the research relationship. Who is being heard in the research and why? The power dynamic in meaning-making processes was explored with reference to real-life examples involving co-operative inquiry into school-based therapy in socially deprived areas, and with reference to the role of black issues in counselling training. In **Chapter 14**, Simon du Plock shared some of his experiences of working as a programme leader for the practice-based research DPsych. Practice-based research takes research out of laboratories and traditional academic settings. What we find in real-life settings will ideally be communicated here too. In this chapter, Simon explores how our research findings can be communicated to a world beyond the university, with those sometimes not used to or already interested in research. In this section, doctoral research is being particularly referred to. For those with an interest in such research, we recommend Goss and Stevens' (2014, in press) *Making Research Matter.*

The value of collegial input and support cannot be emphasised enough. Fortunately, research groups and networks are becoming increasingly accessible. There is, for instance, as Armstrong et al. (2013) conclude, 'a growing interest in Practice Research Networks (PRNs) ... to facilitate practitioner engagement in research and cultivate a more vibrant research culture in the counselling profession'.

Final reflection

You may want to begin to consider if there are any ways of engaging with colleagues or friends about your research? Unless you already belong to a network, the PRNs networks on the BACP website (www.bacp.co.uk) could be a place to start.

Reflexivity involved engaging with other perspectives for long enough to return to a familiar framework with new 'lenses'. Other perspectives can, as Qualley (1997) addressed, be found on different levels and in different places; sometimes within yourself and at other times through others. I would like to take the opportunity to wish you good luck with your discoveries and research, wherever you are looking – and whatever you are looking for!

Recommended reading

Goss, S. and Stevens, C. (2014, in press) *Making Research Matter.* London: Routledge.

This is a collection of real-life examples from psychotherapists working towards their doctorates on a work-based learning programme.

References

Adams, M. (2012) 'Placing ourselves in context: research as personal narrative', in S. Bager-Charleson, *Personal Development in Counselling and Psychotherapy*. London: Learning Matters. pp. 126–37.

Adams, M. (in press) *The Myth of the Untroubled Therapist*. London: Routledge.

Adams-Langley, S. (2011) 'The Place2Be in the Inner City: How Can a Voluntary Sector Mental Health Service have an Impact on Children's Mental Health and the School Environment?' Doctorate in Psychotherapy by Professional Studies, Middlesex University and Metanoia Institute, London.

Aguinaldo, J.P. (2004) 'Rethinking validity in qualitative research from a social constructionist perspective: from "Is this valid research?" to "What is this research valid for?"' *The Qualitative Report*, 9(1), March: 127–36. Available at: www.nova.edu/ssss/QR/QR9-1/aguinaldo.pdf [accessed November 2012].

Alexandrov, H. (2009) 'Experiencing knowledge', in H. Clarke and P. Hodgett (eds), *Researching Beneath the Surface: Psycho-Social Research Methods in Practice*. London: Karnac. pp. 29–51.

Alvesson, M. (2002) *Postmodernism and Social Research*. Buckingham: Open University Press.

Alvesson, M. and Skoldberg, K. (2000) *Reflexive Methodology*. London: Sage.

Argyris, C. and Schön, D. (1974) *Theory in Practise: Increasing Professional Effectiveness*. San Francisco, CA: Jossey-Bass.

Armstrong, J., Hawkins, A. and Thurston, M. (2013) 'Research in practice', *Therapy Today*, 24(4): 35–7.

Asherson Bartram, C. (2009) 'Narratives of Mothers in Stepfamily Situations: An Exploratory Investigation'. Doctorate in Psychotherapy by Professional Studies, Middlesex University and Metanoia Institute, London.

Atkinson, A. (2010) 'The Long-term Post-abortion Experience: What Does a Psychotherapeutic Study Reveal about its Nature and Potential Therapeutic Input'. Doctorate in Psychotherapy, Middlesex University and Metanoia Institute, London.

Aveyard, H. (2010) *Doing a Literature Review in Health and Social Care: A Practical Guide* (2nd edn). Maidenhead: Open University Press.

Aveyard, H. and Sharp, P. (2009) *A Beginner's Guide to Evidence Based Practice in Health and Social Care*. Maidenhead: Open University Press.

BACP (2007) *Ethical Framework for Good Practice in Counselling and Psychotherapy*. Lutterworth: British Association for Counselling and Psychotherapy.

Barber, P. (2006) *Becoming a Practitioner Researcher: A Gestalt Approach to Holistic Inquiry*. London: Middlesex University Press.

Barker, C., Pistrang, N. and Elliott, R. (2002) *Research Methods in Clinical Psychology: An Introduction for Students and Practitioners* (2nd edn). Chichester: John Wiley & Sons.

Barkham, M., Gilbert, N. et al. (2005) 'Suitability and utility of the CORE-OM and CORE-A for assessing severity of presenting problems in psychological therapy services based in primary and secondary care settings', *The British Journal of Psychiatry*, 186: 239–46. Available at: http://bjp.rcpsych.org/content/186/3/239.full [accessed December 2012].

Barkham, M., Hardy, G. and Mellor-Clark, J. (2010) *Developing and Delivering Practice-Based Evidence: A Guide for Psychological Therapies*. Chichester: Wiley-Blackwell.

Beck, A.T., Rush, J., Shaw, B. and Emery, G. (1987) *Cognitive Therapy of Depression*. New York: Guilford Press.

Behar, R. (1996) *The Vulnerable Observer: Anthropology that Breaks Your Heart*. Boston, MA: Beacon Press.

Bell, J. (2010) *Doing Your Research Project: A Guide for First-Time Researchers in Education, Health and Social Science*. Maidenhead: Open University Press.

Bhaskar, R. (1979) *The Possibility of Naturalism: A Philosophical Critique of the Contemporary Human Sciences*. Brighton: Harvester.

Bick, E. (1964) 'Notes on infant observation in psychoanalytic training', *International Journal of Psychoanalysis*, 45(4): 558–66.

Bick, E. (1968) 'The experience of the skin in early object relations', *International Journal of Psychoanalysis*, 49: 484–6.

Bolton, G. (2005) *Reflective Practice: Writing and Professional Development*. London: Sage.

Boote, D.N. and Beile, P. (2005) 'Scholars before researchers: on the centrality of the dissertation literature review in research preparation', *Educational Researcher*, 34(6): 3–15.

Brande, D. (1934/1996) *Becoming a Writer*. London: Macmillan.

Briggs, S. (1997) *Growth and Risk in Infancy*. London: Jessica Kingsley.

Briggs, S. and Behringer, J. (2012) 'Linking infant observation research and other paradigms', in C. Urwin and J. Sternberg (eds), *Infant Observation and Research: Emotional Processes in Everyday Lives*. Hove and New York: Routledge. pp.148–59.

Buber, M. (1958) *I and Thou*. Edinburgh: T. & T. Clarik.

Cameron, J. (1998) *The Right to Write: An Invitation and Initiation into the Writing Life*. London: Pan/Macmillan.

Cardinal, D., Hayward, J. and Jones, G. (2004) *Epistemology: The Theory of Knowledge*. London: Hodder Murray.

Carter, D. and Gradin, S. (2001) *Writing as Reflective Action*. London: Longman.

Chang, H. (2008) *Autoethnography as Method*. Walnut Creek, CA: Left Coast.

Chiari, G. and Nuzzo, M.L. (2010) *Constructivist Psychotherapy: A Narrative Hermeneutic Approach*. London: Taylor & Francis.

Clarke, S. and Hodgett, P. (eds) (2009) *Researching beneath the Surface: Psycho-Social Research Methods in Practice*. London: Karnac.

Clarkson, P. (1995) *The Therapeutic Relationship*. London: Whurr.

Cooper, M. (2003) *Existential Therapies*. London: Sage.

Cooper, M. (2008) *Essential Research Findings*. London: Sage.

Corradi-Fiumara, G. (2001) *The Mind's Affective Life*. Hove: Bunner Routledge.

Costa, B. (2010) 'Mother tongue or non-native language? Learning from conversations with bilingual/multilingual therapists about working with clients who do not share their native language', *Journal of Ethnicity and Inequalities in Health and Social Care*, 3(1): 15–24.

Costa, B. (2012) 'A therapeutic journey across cultural and linguistic borderlands', in S. Bager-Charleson, *Personal Development in Counselling and Psychotherapy*. London: Learning Matters. pp. 137–47.

Costa, B. and Dewaele, J.-M. (2012) 'Psychotherapy across languages: beliefs, attitudes and practices of monolingual and multilingual therapists with their multilingual patients', *Language and Psychoanalysis*, 1: 18–40.

Costley, C., Elliott, G. and Gibbs, P. (2010) *Doing Work-Based Research: Approaches to Enquiry for Insider-Researchers*. London: Sage.

Cottingham, J. (ed.) (2008) *Western Philosophy: An Anthology* (2nd edn). Oxford: Blackwell.

Dancey, C. and Reidy, J. (2011) *Statistics without Maths for Psychology*. Harlow: Pearson-Prentice Hall.

Daniels, M. (2011) 'Using Role Play as a Therapeutic Tool in Offending-Behaviour Programmes in Her Majesty's Prison Service'. Doctorate in Psychotherapy by Professional Studies, Middlesex University and Metanoia Institute, London.

Datler, W., Laxar, R. and Trunkenpolz, K. (2012) 'Observation in nursing home: the use of single case studies and organizational observation as a research tool', in C. Urwin and J. Sternberg (eds), *Infant Observation and Research: Emotional Processes in Everyday Lives*. Hove and New York: Routledge. pp. 160–71.

Dawson, C. (2009) *Introduction to Research Methods* (4th edn). Oxford: How To Books.

Denzin, N. (1989) *Interpretive Interactionism*. Newbury Park, CA: Sage.

Denzin, N. and Lincoln, Y. (2005) *The SAGE Handbook of Qualitative Research*. London: Sage.

Descartes, R. (1641/2008) 'Meditations on first philosophy', in J. Cottingham (ed.), *Western Philosophy: An Anthology* (2nd edn). Oxford: Blackwell. pp. 22–5.

Dewaele, J.-M. (2010) *Emotions in Multiple Languages*. Basingstoke: Palgrave Macmillan.

D'Ombraine Hewitt, R. (2007) *Moving On: A Guide to Good Health and Recovery for People with a Diagnosis of Schizophrenia*. London: Karnac.

D'Ombraine Hewitt, R. (2012) 'Recovery and Transformation: Humanistic-Integrative Counselling and Schizophrenia/Schizo-Affective Disorder: The Client's Perspective'. Middlesex University and Metanoia Institute, London.

Doncaster, K. (2000) 'Recognising and accrediting learning and the development of reflective thinking', in D. Portwood and C. Costey (eds), *Work Based Learning*. Birmingham: SEDA.

Dörnyei, Z. (2007) *Research Methods in Applied Linguistics: Quantitative, Qualitative and Mixed Methodologies*. Oxford: Oxford University Press.

Dörnyei, Z. (2010) *Questionnaires in Second Language Research: Construction, Administration and Processing* (2nd edn). London: Routledge.

du Plock, S. (2005a) '"Silent therapists" and "the community of suffering": some reflections on Bibliotherapy from an existential-phenomenological perspective', *Existential Analysis*, 16 (2): 300–9.

du Plock, S. (2005b) 'Some thoughts on the use of narrative approaches in Counselling Psychology', *Counselling Psychology Review*, 20 (2): 56–65.

du Plock, S. (2006) 'Just what is it that makes contemporary Counselling Psychology so different, so appealing?', *Counselling Psychology Review*, 21 (3): 22–32.

du Plock, S. (2007) 'Using phenomenological research to make a difference: developing a democratic approach to therapeutic reading', *Proceedings of the 25th International Human Science Research Conference: New Frontiers of Phenomenology, beyond Postmodernism in Empirical Research*. Milton Keynes: Open University Press.

du Plock, S. (2010) 'The vulnerable researcher: harnessing reflexivity for practice-based qualitative inquiry', in S. Bager-Charleson (ed.), *Reflective Practice in Counselling and Psychotherapy*. London: Learning Matters.

Edvardsson, D. and Street, A. (2007) 'Sense or no sense: the nurse as embodied ethnographer', *International Journal of Nursing Practice*, 13: 24–32.

Elliott, R. (2002) 'Render unto Caesar: quantitative and qualitative knowing in research on humanistic therapies', *Person-Centered and Experiential Psychotherapies*, 1(1–2): 102–17.

Ellis, C. and Bochner, A. (2000) 'Autoethnography, personal narrative, reflexivity: researcher as subject', in N.K. Norman and Y.S. Denzin (eds), *Handbook of Qualitative Research* (2nd edn). Thousand Oaks, CA: Sage. pp. 733–68.

Etherington, K. (2004) *Becoming a Reflexive Researcher: Using Our Selves in Research*. London: JKP.

Farhady, H. (2013) 'Quantitative methods', in C.A. Chapelle (ed.), *The Encyclopedia of Applied Linguistics*. Oxford: Wiley-Blackwell. pp. 1–8.

Finlay, L. (2012) 'Research: an existential predicament for our profession?', in L. Barnett and G. Madison (eds), *Existential Therapy: Legacy, Vibrancy and Dialogue*. London: Routledge. pp. 183–92.

Finlay, L. and Ballinger, C. (2006) *Qualitative Research for Allied Health Professionals*. Chichester: Wiley.

Finlay, L. and Gough, B. (2003) *Reflexivity: A Practical Guide*. London: Blackwell.

Fishman, D.B. (1999) *The Case for Pragmatic Psychology*. New York and London: New York University.

Fox, M., Martin, P. and Green, G. (2007) *Doing Practitioner Research*. London: Sage.

Freire, P. (1990) *We Make the Road by Walking: Conversations on Education and Social Change*. Philadelphia, PA: Temple University Press.

Freshwater, D. and Lees, J. (2008) *Practitioner-Based Research: Power, Discourse and Transformation*. London: Karnac.

Freud, S. (1900/1976) *The Interpretation of Dreams*. Edited and translated J. Strachey. The Pelican Freud Library, Vol. 4. London: Pelican.

Freud, S. (1922/2008) 'Introductory lectures on psychoanalysis', in J. Cottingham (ed.), *Western Philosophy: An Anthology* (2nd edn). Oxford: Blackwell.

Freud, S. (1940/1959) *An Outline of Psycho-Analysis*. Translated by James Strachey. London: Hogarth Press.

Freud, S. (1997) *The Interpretation of Dreams*. Translated by A.A. Brill. Ware: Wordsworth.

Frith, C. (2007) *Making up the Mind*. Oxford: Blackwell.

Frommer, J. and Langenbach, M. (2001) 'The psychoanalytic case study as a source of epistemic knowledge', in G. Bäumler (ed.), *Qualitative Psychotherapy: Research and Methodology*. Munich: Pabst Science Publishers. pp. 508–26.

Gardner, F. (2006) 'Using critical reflection in research and evaluation', in S. White, J. Fook and F. Gardner (eds), *Critical Reflection in Health and Social Care*. Maidenhead: Open University Press. pp. 144–55.

Giacomini, M. (2001) 'The rocky road: qualitative research as evidence – EBM notebook', *Evidence Based Medicine*, 6: 4–6. Available at: http://ebm.bmj.com/content/6/1/4.full [accessed November 2012].

Gilbert, P. and Leahy, R. (eds) (2007) *The Therapeutic Relationship in the Cognitive Behavioural Psychotherapies*. London: Routledge.

Goss, S.P. (2002) *Counselling: A Quiet Revolution*. London: Teachers' Benevolent Fund.

Goss, S.P. and Mearns, D. (1997) 'Applied pluralism in the evaluation of employee counselling', *British Journal of Guidance and Counselling*, 25(3): 189–98.

Goss, S.P. and Stevens, C. (2014, in press) *Making Research Matter*. London: Routledge.

Graves, N. and Varma, V. (eds) (1999) *Working for a Doctorate: A Guide for the Humanities and Social Sciences*. London: Routledge.

Greco, J. and Sosa, E. (1999) *Blackwell Guide Epistemology* (Blackwell Philosophy Guides). Oxford: Blackwell.

Haraway, D.J. (1991) *Simians, Cyborgs, and Women: The Reinvention of Nature*. London: Free Association.

Hatch, E. and Farhady, H. (1982) *Research Design and Statistics for Applied Linguistics*. New York: Newbury House.

Heron, J. (1996) *Cooperative Inquiry: Research into the Human Condition*. London: Sage.

Hiles, D. (2001) 'Heuristic inquiry and transpersonal research'. Leicester: Psychology Department, De Montfort University. Available at: www.psy.dmu.ac.uk/drhiles/HIpaper.htm [accessed November 2012].

Hinshelwood, R.D. (1997) 'Psychodynamic formulation in assessment for psychoanalytic psychotherapy', in C. Mace (ed.), *The Art and Science of Assessment in Psychotherapy*. London: Routledge.

Hinshelwood, R.D. and Skogstadt, W. (2000) *Observing Organisations: Anxiety, Defence and Culture in Health Care*. London and New York: Routledge.

Hoffman, T., Bennett, S. and Del Mar, C. (eds) (2009) *Evidence-Based Practice across the Health Professions*. Chatswood: Elsevier.

Hollway, W. (2011) 'In between external and internal worlds: imagination in transitional space', *Methodological Innovations Online*, 6(3): 50–60. Available at: www.pbs.plym.ac.uk/mi/pdf/8-02-12/MIO63Paper23.pdf [accessed December 2012].

Hollway, W. and Jefferson, T. (2000) *Doing Qualitative Research Differently*. London: Sage.

Hollway, W. and Jefferson, T. (2012) *Doing Qualitative Research Differently* (2nd edn). London: Sage.

Hopkins, M.J. (2012) 'Staff Experience of Hope in a Forensic Psychiatric Hospital'. Doctorate in Psychotherapy by Professional Studies, Middlesex University and Metanoia Institute, London.

Husserl, E. (1960/1999) 'Cartesian meditations', in M. Friedman (ed.), *The Worlds of Existentialism: A Critical Reader*. New York: Humanity Books. pp. 77–83.

Josselson, R. (2011) '"Bet you think this song is about you": whose narrative is it in narrative research?', *Fielding Graduate University*, 1(1). Available at: Journals.hil.unb.ca/index.php/NW/article/download/18472/ 19971 [accessed 21 November 2012].

Josselson, R. (2013) *Interviewing for Qualitative Inquiry: A Relational Approach*. New York and London: Guilford Press.

Kandel, E. (2006) *In Search of Memory*. New York: W.W. Norton.

Kant, I. (1783/2008) 'Prolegomena', in J. Cottingham (ed.), *Western Philosophy: An Anthology* (2nd edn). Oxford: Blackwell, pp. 108–14.

Kant, I. (1787/2007) *Critique of Pure Reason*. Translated by Marcus Wiegelt. London: Penguin.

Karamati Ali, R. (2004) 'Bilingualism and systemic psychotherapy: some formulations and explorations', *Journal of Family Therapy*, 26: 340–57.

Kasket, E. (2012) 'The counselling psychologist researcher', *Counselling Psychology Review*, 27(2): 64–73.

Kim-Cohen, J., Caspi, A., Moffitt, T.E., Harrington, H., Milne, B.J. and Poulton, R. (2003) *Prior Juvenile Diagnoses in Adults with Mental Disorder: Developmental Follow-back of a Prospective-longitudinal Cohort*. London: Institute of Psychiatry, King's College. Available at: www.ncbi.nlm.nih.gov/pubmed/12860775

Kolb, D.A. (1984) *Experiential Learning*. London: Prentice Hall.

Langridge, D. (2007) *Phenomenological Psychology*. Harlow: Pearson.

Lee, N.J. (2009) *Achieving Your Professional Doctorate: A Handbook*. Milton Keynes: Open University Press.

Leech, N.L. and Dellinger, A. (2013) 'Validity: mixed methods', in C.A. Chapelle (ed.), *The Encyclopedia of Applied Linguistics*. Oxford: Wiley-Blackwell. pp. 1–7.

Lewin, K. (1952) *Field Theory in Social Science: Selected Papers*. London: Tavistock.

Livholts, M. (ed.) (2013) *Emergent Writing Methodologies in Feminist Studies*. London: Routledge.

Marks, D.F. (2002) *Perspectives on Evidence-based Practice*. [Online]. Department of Psychology, City University, London, and Health Development Agency. Available at: www.nice.org.uk/niceMedia/pdf/persp_ evid_dmarks.pdf [accessed 1 December 2012].

Masten, A., Best, K. and Garmezy, N. (1990) 'Resilience and development: contributions from the study of children who overcome adversity', *Developmental Psychopathology*, 2: 425–44.

Mckenzie-Mavinga, I. (2005) 'A Study of Black Issues in Counsellor Training 2002–2005'. Doctorate in Psychotherapy by Professional Studies, Middlesex University and Metanoia Institute, London.

McLeod, J. (1994) *Doing Counselling Research*. London: Sage.

McLeod, J. (1999) *Practitioner Research in Counselling*. London: Sage.

McLeod, J. (2001) *Qualitative Research in Counselling and Psychotherapy*. London: Sage.

McLeod, J. (2012) 'Systematic Case Study Research in Psychotherapy: Principles and Methods'. University of Abertay, Dundee, John Tayside Institute for Health Studies. Available at: www.crfr.ac.uk/reports/JMcleod.pdf [accessed 15 December 2012].

McLeod, J. (2013) *An Introduction to Research in Counselling and Psychotherapy*. London: Sage.

McLeod, T. (ed.) (1987) *Collins Concise Dictionary of the English Language*. London: Guild Publishing.

Messer, S.B. (2004) 'Evidence-based practice: beyond empirically supported treatments', *Professional Psychology: Research and Practice*, 35: 580–8.

Miell, D. and Dallos, R. (1996) *Social Interaction and Personal Relationships*. London: Sage.

Morris, G.H. and Chenail, R.J. (1994) *The Talk Clinic: Explorations in the Analysis of Medical and Therapeutic Discourse*. Abingdon: Routledge.

Moule, P. and Hek, G. (2011) *Making Sense of Research*. London: Sage.

Moustakas, C. (1990) *Heuristic Research: Design, Methodology and Applications*. London: Sage.

Moustakas, C. (1994) *Phenomenological Research Methods*. London: Sage.

Mullins, G. and Kiley, M. (2002) '"It's a PhD, not a Nobel prize": how experienced examiners assess research theses', *Studies in Higher Education*, 27(4): 369–86.

Muncey, T. (2010) *Creating Autoethnography*. London: Sage.

Neuhaus, E.C. (2011) 'Becoming a cognitive-behavioral therapist: striving to integrate professional and personal development', in R. Klein, H.S. Bernard and V. Schermer (eds), *On Becoming a Psychotherapist: The Personal and Professional Journey*. Oxford and New York: Oxford University Press. pp. 212–44.

Nguyen, B. (2012) 'Working with Monolingual and Bilingual Clients in the UK when English is not your First Language'. Unpublished MA Dissertation, Reading University, UK.

NICE (2007) *Depression (Amended): Management of Depression in Primary and Secondary Care*. London: National Institute for Health and Clinical Excellence.

Parker, I. (1994) 'Qualitative research', in I. Parker, P. Banister, E. Burman, M. Taylor and C. Tindall, *Qualitative Methods in Psychology*. Buckingham: Open University Press.

Parker, I. (2007) *Revolution in Psychology*. London: Pluto Press.

Parker, I., Banister, P., Burman, E., Taylor, M. and Tindall, C. (1994) *Qualitative Methods in Psychology*. Buckingham: Open University Press.

Pink, S. (2009) *Doing Sensory Ethnography*. London: Sage.

Pistrang, N. and Barker, C. (2010) 'Scientific, practical and personal dimensions in selecting qualitative methods', in M. Barkham, G. Hardy and J. Mellor-Clark (eds), *Developing and Delivering Practice-Based Evidence: A Guide for Psychological Therapies*. Chichester: Wiley-Blackwell. pp. 65–90.

Popper, K. (1957/2008) 'Science and falsifiability: conjectures and refutation', in J. Cottingham (ed.), *Western Philosophy: An Anthology* (2nd edn). Oxford: Blackwell. pp. 453–60.

Price, H. and Cooper, A. (2012) 'In the field: psychoanalytic observation and epistemological realism', in C. Urwin and J. Sternberg (eds), *Infant Observation and Research: Emotional Processes in Everyday Lives*. Hove and New York: Routledge. pp. 55–67.

Priest, A. (2013) 'You and I Listening to Me: Towards an Understanding of the Significance of Personal Pronoun Usage in Psychotherapy'. Doctorate in Psychotherapy, Middlesex University and Metanoia Institute, London.

Qualley, D. (1997) *Turns of Thought*. Portsmouth: Boynton/Cook Heinemann.

Racker, H. (2001) *Transference and Countertransference*. London: Karnac.

Reason, P. (1994) *Participation in Human Inquiry*. London: Sage.

Ricoeur, P. (1970) *Freud and Philosophy: An Essay on Interpretation*. Translated D. Savage. New Haven, CT, and London: Yale University Press.

Robson, C. (2002) *Real World Research* (2nd edn). Oxford: Blackwell.

Rogers, C. (1951) *Client-centred Therapy*. London: Constable.

Rogers, C. (1961) *A Therapist's View of Psychotherapy*. London: Constable & Co.

Rogers, C. (1995) *A Way of Being*. New York: Houghton Mifflin.

Rosen, H. and Kuehlwein, K.T. (eds) (1996) *Constructing Realities*. San Francisco, CA: Jossey-Bass.

Sackett, D.L. et al. (2000) *Evidence-Based Medicine: How to Practice and Teach EBM* (2nd edn). London: Churchill Livingstone.

Sanders, P. and Wilkins, P. (2010) *First Steps in Practitioner Research*. Ross-on-Wye: PCCS Books.

Scaife, J. (2001) 'The contracting process and the supervisory relationship', in J. Scaife (ed.), *In Supervision in the Mental Health Professions: A Practitioner's Guide*. Hove: Brunner Routledge. Chapter 4, pp. 52–69.

Schön, D.A. (1983) *The Reflective Practitioner*. New York: Basic Books.

Schore, A.N. (2003) 'The human unconscious: the development of the right brain and its role in the early emotional life', in V. Greene (ed.), *Emotional Development in Psychoanalysis, Attachment Theory and Neuroscience*. Brighton: Routledge. pp. 23–54.

Sedgwick, D. (1994) *The Wounded Healer: Countertransference from a Jungian Perspective*. London: Routledge.

Shuttleworth, J. (2012) 'Infant observation, ethnography and social anthropology', in C. Urwin and J. Sternberg (eds), *Infant Observation and Research: Emotional Processes in Everyday Lives*. Hove and New York: Routledge. pp. 171–81.

Slevin, O. (2001) 'An epistemology of nursing: ways of knowing and being', in L. Basford and O. Slevin, *Theory and Practice Nursing: An Integrative Approach to Caring Practice*. Cheltenham: Nelson Thorne. pp. 143–72.

Smith, F. (1991) *Writing and the Writer* (2nd edn). Englewood Cliffs, NJ: Laurence Erlbaum Associates.

Smith, J.A. (2004) 'Reflecting on the development of interpretative phenomenological analysis and its contribution to qualitative psychology', *Qualitative Research in Psychology*, 1: 39–54.

Smith, J.A., Flowers, P. and Larkin, M. (2009) *Interpretive Phenomenological Analysis: Theory, Method, and Research*. London: Sage.

Solms, M. and Turnbull, O. (2002) *The Brain and the Inner World*. London: Karnac.

Souter-Andersson, L. (2011) 'Exploring the Use of Clay as Therapy: Towards a Formulation of a Theoretical Model'. Doctoral project, Middlesex University and Metanoia Institute, London.

Spence, D.P. (1989) 'Rhetoric vs. evidence as source of persuasion: a critique of the case study genre', in M.J. Packer and R.B. Addison (eds), *Entering the Circle*. New York: State University of New York Press. pp. 205–21.

Spencer, L. (2006) 'Tutors' stories of personal development training: attempting to maximise learning potentials', *Counselling and Psychotherapy Research*, 6(2): 108–14.

Stanley, M. (2006) 'A grounded theory of the wellbeing of older people', in L. Finlay and C. Ballinger (eds), *Qualitative Research for Allied Health Professionals: Challenging Choices*. Chichester: Wiley. pp. 63–78.

Stewart, P. (1998) 'Born Inside: An Observational Study of Mothers and Babies in Holloway Prison'. MA dissertation, Tavistock Clinic/University of East London.

Stiles, W.B. (2010) 'Theory-building case studies as practice-based evidence', in M. Barkham, G. Hardy and J. Mellor-Clark (eds), *Developing and Delivering Practice-Based Evidence: A Guide for Psychological Therapies*. Chichester: Wiley-Blackwell. pp. 91–109.

Strauss, A. and Corbin, J. (2008) *Basics of Qualitative Research: Techniques and Procedures for Developing Grounded Theory*. Thousand Oaks, CA: Sage.

Stuart, C. and Whitmore, E. (2008) 'Using reflexivity in a research methods course: bridging the gap between research and practice', in S. White, J. Fook and F. Gardner (eds), *Critical Reflection in Health and Social Care*. Maidenhead: Open University Press. pp. 156–71.

Symington, N. (1986) *The Analytic Experience*. London: Free Association.

Tashakkori, A. and Teddlie, C. (eds) (2010) *Handbook of Mixed Methods in Social and Behavioral Research*. Thousand Oaks, CA: Sage.

Thompson, K. (2011) *Therapeutic Journal Writing: An Introduction for Professionals*. London and Philadelphia, PA: Jessica Kingsley.

Teddlie, C. and Tashakkori, A. (2009) *Foundations of Mixed Methods Research: Integrating Quantitative and Qualitative Approaches in the Social and Behavioral Sciences*. Thousand Oaks, CA: Sage.

Trahar, S. (2009) 'Beyond the story itself: narrative inquiry and autoethnography in intercultural research in higher education' [41 paragraphs], *Forum: Qualitative Sozialforschung / Forum: Qualitative Social Research*, 10(1), Art. 30. Available at: www.qualitative-research.net/index.php/fqs/article/view/ 1218/2653.

UK Council for Graduate Education (2002) *Professional Doctorates* [online]. Available at: www.uhr.no/documents/ProfessionalDoctorates2002.pdf [accessed 13 December 2012].

University of California Santa Cruz (n.d.) *Write a Literature Review* [online]. Available at: www.guides.library.ucsc.edu/write-a-literature-review [accessed 24 November 2012].

Urwin, C. and Sternberg, J. (2012) *Infant Observation and Research: Emotional Processes in Everyday Lives*. Hove & New York: Routledge.

Van Deurzen, E. and Arnold-Baker, C. (2005) *Existential Perspectives on Human Issues: A Handbook for Therapeutic Practice*. London: Palgrave Macmillan.

Warburton, N. (2004) *Philosophy: The Basics*. Abingdon: Routledge.

Welldon, E. (1991) *Mother, Madonna, Whore: The Idealization and Denegration of Motherhood*. London: Karnac.

Wengraf, T. (2001) *Qualitative Research Interviewing*. London: Sage.

Wheeler, S. and Elliott, R. (2008) 'What do counsellors and psychotherapists need to know about research?', *Counselling and Psychotherapy Research*, 8(2): 133–5.

White, S., Fook, J. and Gardner, F. (eds) (2006) *Critical Reflection in Health and Social Care*. Maidenhead: Open University Press.

Whittaker, A. (2009) *Research Skills for Social Work*. Exeter: Learning Matters.

Wilson, R. and Dewaele, J.-M. (2010) 'The use of web questionnaires in second language acquisition and bilingualism research', *Second Language Research*, 26: 103–23.

Winnicott, D.W. (1961) *The Maturational Processes and the Facilitating Environment*. London: Karnac.

Winter, R., Buck, A. and Sobiechowska, P. (1999) *Professional Experience and the Investigative Imagination: The Art of Reflective Writing*. London: Routledge.

Yalom, I.D. (1980) *Existential Psychotherapy*. New York: Basic Books.

Yalom, I.D. (1991) *Love's Executioner and Other Tales of Psychotherapy*. London: Penguin.

Yalom, I.D. (2002) *The Gift of Therapy*. London: Piatkus.

Yorks, L. and Kasl, E. (2002) 'Learning from the inquiries: lessons for using collaborative inquiry as an adult learning strategy', *New Directions for Adult and Continuing Education*, 94: 93–104.

Index